Diary of a Diet:
A Little Book of Big

Hannah Jones

Published by Accent Press Ltd – 2007
ISBN 190612504X/ 9781906125042
Copyright © Hannah Jones and The Western Mail 2007

Printed and bound in the UK

Cover Design and Photography by
Darryl Corner

About The Author

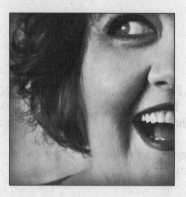

Hannah Jones is Magazine Editor for the Western Mail, the National Newspaper of Wales. A Valleys girl from Ebbw Vale, she is a Philosophy graduate with a couple of musical Grade 8s to her name.

She became a journalist when her Top of the Pops dreams failed to materialize and her operatic skills were in danger of being noticed.

She has since made an album nobody has heard of and the only remnant of her classical training remaining is an ability to sound convincing when ordering food at an Italian restaurant. She lives near Caerphilly and *Diary of a Diet* is her first book.

www.hannahjones.net

For anyone who's ever weighed
out their chips

(or themselves)

Acknowledgments

Darryl Corner, for everything and then some. Jonathan Amphlett, aka Hiya Love, my housemate, champion swede masher and general superstar. The girls at work – Karen Price, Cathryn Scott, Saffron Jenkins, Ceri Gould, Louise Robjohn, Claire Hill, Rin Simpson, Madeleine Brindley, Jacky Thomas and the front counter gang – who never stopped laughing and supporting the cause. Nicola Giles, who's always attempted to get me a proper 'G' for Good (and not just a grade in Biology) in everything I do. Julian Meek and Marc White, fast-fingered visionaries in their own unique ways. Samantha Jones, it's a pleasure knowing you and working alongside you. And the big boss, Alan Edmunds, for simply saying Yes.

But most of all this book is in full-fat gratitude to Sophie and John Jones, my mam and dad. They always believed.

Foreword

The reason I go on about my weight in my act is because everybody else bloody does too.

As a woman you are almost totally defined in our society by your appearance, so woe betide if you are a fat woman; your personality, history, opinions, ambitions will all be hidden under the never-changing critical eye of men and women who don't struggle with their weight and just see you as a blob.

Refuse to be that blob – be irritating, be rude, be annoying, but don't just be a blob.

To do comedy you just have to be funny and so whether you are fat or thin isn't important.

An audience will tell you if they like you by laughing and thank the Lord for me, they did.

But most women's lives are an endless struggle against their ever-rising weight.

I know what it's like, it's tragic – so you might as well have a fucking laugh about it.

Jo Brand

> **Fat: adjective; affording good opportunities, esp. for gain; of major concern, importance, gravity, or the like**

IT SOUNDED LIKE A good idea at the time.

Waved in front of me was a gym membership at a fancy hotel and a washboard-bellied personal trainer who'd willingly let me smash him in the face with pink boxing gloves twice a week.

All I had to do in return was write about the trials and tribulations of trying to get fit AND lose weight (there's a laugh) every Tuesday.

In their wisdom, the sages at the *Western Mail*, the fancily titled National Newspaper of Wales where I work as Magazine Editor, decided to call these columns of mine 'Diary of a Diet'.

It felt to me like the kind of place where I could bare my soul (luckily not my stomach or love(less) handles) for the nation to see, somewhere where these confessions of mine would spur me into activity. You can't hide in print, can you? Especially when your mother is reading.

That was a year and a half ago and this book is my account of the time.

If you're anything like me, you will have been on countless diets, self-medicated with carbs, judged yourself by your waist size and not the girth of your IQ, achievements or how bloody nice you are, and

1

wondered if you'd ever get to grips with yourself, that authentic (thank you Oprah) part of you that wakes up EVERY morning – and not just 1 in 77 – and screams, bugger it, you're fabulous just the way you are. And that doesn't matter if you're a size 8 or a 28.

Anyway, so there I was, armed with nothing but a lifetime of skewed thinking about my allure and size, not so much running towards this challenge of sharing my failures with the nation (because that's how I saw it) as doing a mild saunter in its direction.

At least I felt qualified – hey, I'd tried the Atkins, the egg diet, two cabbage ones, the fat free thingie, Slimming World, WeightWatchers – online and off – Rosemary C and the GI.

I'd even given Abject Misery a go, thinking that maybe public dieting would slim me down and thereby make my self-esteem fatter.

Nothing had really worked before. And, frankly, at 34 I was desperate to see my toes without acting like some fat-arsed circus freak who looked liked she was a model for the makers of Fun House mirrors, AFTER you'd gone in, not before.

So I looked at writing 'Diary of a Diet' as a kind of open letter to myself, being as frank as I could, revealing my own personal truth in the most brutal of ways and also getting the chance to stick two éclair-like fingers up at the diet industry (I know, I know…) and shove my wide fitting, high hells (sic) avoiding, size 7s right into the fat-free heart of the Size Zero debate.

For the record, the column wasn't started by someone who needed to drop ONE dress size or tone up A BIT.

When it began I was at least seven stone overweight and a size 24. Go on, read that again. Slowly.

The difference between me and most women, though, is that I have never harboured ambitions to be a size 12.

I'm just a normal someone who'd like to fit into a size 18-20 dress (Christ, now there's a thing…) and think, finally, that what I feel on the outside is doing what I'm capable of on the inside justice.

I was just fed up with feeling fat, with, in internet terms at least, being more niche market than marketable as a sexy, sassy, sorted, strong woman.

In the column, much of which you'll find in this book along with other size related musings, I've talked about my relationship with food (complex, unlike the healthiest kind of carbs I'm told), denial (it's not just a river in Egypt where fat people go to wash away their troubles you know), exercise (if I'd been built to bend, there'd be pork pies with crispy crusts on the floor as a reward) and fat being the most effective contraceptive (why even big buggers like me can say No to men who aren't so much fattist as blind to the notion of big, big love).

I've gone into detail about the diets I've loved to hate and not lost anything on, about reaching for food when people have disappointed me (go on, tell me you've *never* hunted down a family-sized bar of

Fruit & Nut while trying to make sense of it all, whatever your size), how ridiculously sensitive I am to criticism, and how frankly crap I am at judging my own attractiveness and worth.

So if you're looking for a proper diet book, for pages and pages on what to eat and at what time to optimise weight loss, you'll be disappointed. This isn't that kind of reading because you can do it while dipping chocolate digestives in full fat frothy coffee.

It's simply the story of me, someone who wishes they were more than they are (but not in the boob/thigh ratio department, thank you very much); it's a book about being big but sometimes feeling small, of what I feel when I hear perfectly proportioned thinnies drone on about their Size Zero fantasies. It's a book about the very ordinary act of living in this stretched-beyond-reason skin right now.

And, talking to women who've commented about it every week – fat, thin, tubby, perfect – it seems it's also about their battles too.

So here I am. Literally at the start of a new chapter of a book, and some very meaty questions still remain.

Have I lost weight?

Do I look in the mirror and feel satisfied?

Am I still shopping at Evans for giant sized smalls?

Do I perceive myself as being so fat, I still get stuck in my own dreams?

Do I feel like a fat-arsed cheerleader for all

women, a pale imitation of Tyra Banks who'll bang on about accepting yourself just the way you are?

Will I ever manage to get a bra that fits?

Will I finally accept that I'm just wonderful, as I am today, right this minute?

Do I reveal by the end of the book what I weigh? And does it really matter anyway?

I'm not a thinker, an arguer, a philosopher or a feminist. I'm just someone who's weak around corned beef rolls and cheese and onion pasties and has spent a lifetime wishing she wasn't. I'm also someone who isn't afraid to admit my weaknesses.

It takes a lot of unravelling to work out how we see ourselves, even if you're one of those lucky sods who can tuck a crisp white shirt into skinny jeans while doing it (and to realise that desserts spelled backwards is stressed).

This, for me then, is just the beginning – yet another one.

Hannah Jones

> **Any people whose lives are about the way they look, whether it's fat or thin, are in a dangerous area**
>
> **Dawn French**

IT'S GOING TO HAPPEN tomorrow.

Whenever it's happened before, it's always been on a Monday because I've convinced myself good things should start at the beginning of the week. Hey, maybe it's an omen. Then again, maybe not.

I've lost count of how many 'fresh starts' I've had in my 34 years, how many Mondays I've seen which I thought would hold the golden 24 hours when I'd finally do something about being my own worst enemy.

These mystical Mondays were total nonsense of course, hope-filled days turning more swiftly into more ordinary days, where Tuesdays became synonymous with failure. And Tuesdays aren't Mondays, are they?

And you know the rule, girls – if you're gonna change your life/your thinking/take the C out of Chips and make it into svelte Hips, you've got to do it on a Monday. Or so I thought.

Tomorrow is Wednesday, the day where I *could* start to become a new, healthier, happier Hannah. Technically speaking at least.

Tomorrow is the day where I embarrass myself into action and put my insecurities, my unease with myself, my internal nonsense on the line for you to see.

It's the day where I join a gym and ask you to watch me as I fail, flail, struggle, sweat, get frustrated, get annoyed, get pissed off with myself and my inability to stick at anything; it's the first day of getting back my sense of self.

There's this advert on the telly at the mo plugging some new magazine that looks at women's twisted thinking about their bodies and concept of attractiveness.

Some fancy voice-over girl with marbles in her mouth asks, "Are you unhappy because of your weight, or do you have a problem with your weight because you are unhappy?" or some such complicated psychobabble.

That's like asking, "If there's no one to watch me eating a crisp sandwich, does it really happen?"

If I could stand up in a circle before you all I'd tell you, "Hello, my name's Hannah and I'm fat and lazy. I need help, I need encouragement, I need support and I need to try and get healthy or I feel I'll just close in on myself and give up trying to be a better version of the work in progress that is me."

Because I can't hide here, can I?

This is as open as it gets ladies and gents, and this is going to be my truth. So tomorrow at 11am, I'm off to a hotel where there's a swanky new gym and men and women in tight clothing with big smiles who will tell me, in a nice way, "Yep, you're a lumper all right." And I'm dreading it.

For the record, because this isn't going to be a column written by someone who needs to drop a dress size or has the tiniest bulge in her belly like she's eaten a Malteser, I'm at least seven stone over weight.

I won't tell you what I weigh, but I will tell you that I'm just a normal someone who'd like to fit into a size 18 dress.

Maybe then I'd think, finally, what I feel on the outside is doing what I'm capable of on the inside justice.

Yes, tomorrow is Wednesday… and it just could be the Monday of my new life.

> # I don't exercise. If God wanted me to bend over, he'd have put diamonds on the floor
>
> **Joan Rivers**

I'M A MINOR CELEBRITY. Scratch that, I'm a fat minor celebrity.

In the two weeks I've been writing my 'Diary of a Diet' column, I've had a book sent in asking me 'Why Do You Overeat?' (thanks Zoë Harcombe), emails from strangers urging me to keep up the good work (while obviously hoping I don't eat chunky KitKats for breakfast – sorry, I succumbed yesterday morning), and people coming up to me and chatting about weight loss in general.

And these are people I've never met before, people who know of me because of my job at the Western Mail and not because I've admitted to being a lazy over-eater.

But do you know what? Their concern, their smiles, their empathy honestly make me think I'm not alone in this big – and bloody hell, it is big – battle of wills.

Fat or thin – and most of them are what I would class as 'small' – it seems we're all obsessed with our body image and chopsing together about what we can do about it.

I have a new best friend, Abs, whom I can confide in, though. I met him last week, and for two hours he talked at me about life, love, the universe and everything to do with being fat.

He avoided directly using the 'F' word though,

sometimes replacing it with that little chestnut 'unhappy', but he didn't dodge the issue. And, frankly, he's fit enough to jump over it.

It was on Wednesday, and he sent me packing from the hotel's new 'lifestyle' spa in Cardiff with homework and the promise that I'd keep a food diary.

I've done the shock therapy treatment part of the deal where I become a pseudo-American and write down how I feel, what I look like, what I think people think I look like, why I need to change – and what a jumble of self-deluded nonsense that was. But, hey, it's *my* deluded nonsense and it's my twisted version of reality.

I haven't done the food diary though, rather I've kept tabs on how many times I took the stairs as opposed to the lift in work (twice in a week); if I walked the dog for half an hour a day (Bertie, I'm so, so, *so* sorry, love), or if I felt that I was on the road to what the AAers call Recovery (umm... nope, don't think so. And I don't think I'd recognise it if it sat next to me covered in cheese in Pizza Hut).

I don't know why I haven't kept a food diary, cataloguing what I already know – that I don't eat breakfast and that I sometimes don't eat or drink a thing for about 13 hours at a time.

Or that conversely I can eat enough breakfast for an army and binge like there's no tomorrow or next week.

I'm ready for my first proper work-out with Abs tomorrow, where there's less talk, more action, and the looming threat of my becoming seriously depressed about letting myself become so sluggish.

I can feel the frustration jabbing at me already. I just hope big, fit, strong, wonderful and wise Abs is man enough to know a woman in need is a woman as fragile as glass and cripplingly insecure.

He'll also need to know that during these times we all think that life's a bitch.

And so am I.

Beware of all enterprises that require new clothes

Henry David Thoreau

YOU'VE GOT TO LOOK the part, right?

A quick trawl through my mental filing cabinet and I see it's been an OK week.

I met with Abs, the long limbed wise man also known as my personal trainer on Wednesday for our first proper work out.

It all started well enough… until I got to the spa. Ah, the semantics of being fat – it's not easy being a lumper, you know.

A burning depression started to stab at me as soon as I got in the dressing room and took out my new gym gear.

No pastel all-in-one sheath for me – I'd gone into Oompa Loompa Girl and got myself kitted out with clothes that I thought looked big enough to contain me without restraining me.

And as I pulled on the trousers, the downward spiral started – too short in the leg, therefore too short in the body leaving me looking like I was wearing a body harness and someone had shoved me out of a plane. It looked as if I had an open burger and bap sandwich thing going on down below, if you know what I mean.

The top was so short it could have doubled as a bolero jacket. I stood there in ill-fitting gear, my work blouse underneath it all to at least give me some semblance of dignity.

Luckily for me, Abs doesn't give a flying pedometer what I look like. All he cares about is encouraging me to be better than I am, fitter than I am, stronger than I am.

I didn't bother telling him my frustration levels were at an all time high, primarily because I felt like the love child of Wallace and Gromit – ugly, stilted and wearing the wrong trousers.

Abs, literally pulling me up by my trousers as I balanced precariously on a big ball while stretching bits of me that didn't want to give, didn't care about my inner turmoil or trouser trouble, though.

He coaxed me into accessing another place, a fantasy island where my trousers not only fitted but were at least three sizes smaller.

And to get there he took me cycling, walking and, wearing a pair of pink luminous gloves, boxing.

BOXING! It was the most fun I've had with my clothes on this side of the 12th of Never. Pink-gloved hand on uncertain heart, I loved my first session with Abs, the encouraging emails that followed, the little texts saying "well done", not to mention the tongue-in-cheek tips on how to dispose of pizza boxes ("have Chinese instead... the cartons are easier to ball up and throw away"). But I haven't been back to the gym since Wednesday.

I'm not sure why, but left to my own devices I lack resolve, and this keeps me where I am. Pushed, prodded and poked by someone else with my best intentions at heart, I'm much better.

The good news is that I have, however, increased what Abs calls my 'inactivity activity' (basically walking up the stairs in work and not taking the lift up a flight), I ate breakfast and, to cap it all, I have my bag filled with my other set of exercise clothes packed and nestled next to me under my desk, ready for the moment to strike.

The rest, as Abs would say, is all up to me.

But somehow I really wish that it wasn't.

Forget love – I'd rather fall in chocolate

Anonymous

"I THINK HE'S INTO that stuff you used to like. What's it called now? Betty the Vegetable Slayer I think," my man friend tells me.

(Vegetables. I'm so hungry I'd even consider some.)

"Then he put on this film called Disappearance. So he asked me if I'd seen it, right?

"And I don't want to tell him I haven't... you know me, I can't sit through a bath, let alone a film.

"So anyway I thought, right buttie, time to think on your feet. So I told him I'd seen it and liked it. You know, just so I don't look like a complete culture victim.

"And he goes to me, 'If you like it, what's it about then?'

"Oh shit," I think to myself. And then it comes to me.

"'It's about a magician'. It's about a bloody murder, isn't it!"

(I could murder a sandwich. How long is it since I had a sandwich? About four months I think. And then it was on thin-see-ya bread.)

"So we sit through the film, bloody disturbing it was too, and he tells me what he does for a living. He's a medical rep. Well, not really a rep."

(I wonder if I have a reputation in the office for being

*a compulsive overeater? I wonder if I'm talked about in
loos and canteens and during fag breaks? There's a girl
downstairs who drinks her cereal milk, slurping it out of
a bowl after she's finished her Crunchy Nuts. They all
talk about her.)*

"What he does, right, is make prosthetic limbs. Don't
laugh! Well, not make them – he's not much good with
plaster of Paris, he says, but I'm not sure if he was
having me on. Anyway, I think he's got all his own arms
and legs – I'd have bloody died if he took his leg off for
me to see! I think he's armless anyway. Get it? Armless.
Ha!"

*(I could do with new legs. And arms. And ears. Maybe a
nose, as I think mine looks like Dad's. And he was a
boxer. "You've got your father's nose and back", is
Mam's mantra. I wish I had his strength of character. I
wonder if this new fella does false hope by the box?)*

"And he's got his nipple pierced. I said I wasn't fussed
on that, but I didn't mind really. So I told him I had
tattoos on my back. Red or Dead, I said – that's what's
on there. Only I got it a bit wrong. That's the make of
your glasses isn't it? Shit. What I meant to say was Love
and Hate, you know, so I'd look hard. I didn't, of course,
mention the fact that the one time I went to get one done
I fainted in the waiting room. Or that I have to have gas
and air at the dentist's."

*(Gas. I think I've got gas. I wonder if it's a hang over
from my Atkins days? And my hair's terrible. Should I
buy big knickers? Those ones like a girdle. Maybe my
skinny jeans would fit then. Sam from work said she*

17

bought a pair to wear under this dress. But it was so tight she was afraid to fart in case she burped. Who'd care though? She's shaped like an egg timer, filled with grains of glamour that never seem to run out of steam. She could blow off and no bugger would care. Me? I'd blow a hole through the ozone layer if I cut the cheese, as those eloquent Americans say.)

"And I told him all about you, said what you do for a living, said how funny you are, how pretty, how close we are, how you're on a diet."

(Is that all there is to me? Sentences which stop at 'diet'? Does it define me? That reminds me, I'm bloody starving.)

"Want to watch a DVD? He let me borrow a couple of real crackers he had for Christmas. Said I could have them back the next time I see him."

(Crackers. I'd eat them without cheese because I only like cheese if it's melted. Crackers with crackers please, for Miss Crackers. Why didn't I have any chocolates for Christmas? In fact, there was a decided lack of chocolate anywhere in the house now that I come to think of it. And the only DVD I had was that fitness one by that girl who won Skating on Ice. Gaynor Faye was it? You know, her off Fat Friends. *Why don't I have any fat friends? You know what they say, if you want to look thin you should hang around with fat people. Where the hell does that leave me? Looking fatter? Nicola's tiny, Karen's a 12 up the top and 14 down the bottom, Lou's normal apart from her gloriously fully ripened melon-shaped globes of joy, Sam's perfection with wild hair, Ceri's a perfect size*

*10 or maybe 8, Jacky's a high-heeled 12 I'd say. Maybe
they're hanging out with me for the wrong reasons. Oh
shit. You think so? Nah, it's because I don't exercise
portion control (or exercise at all in fact) when they
come round for supper. They never have seconds though.
Wonder if that has anything to do with the sight of me,
usually bra-less and feeling hopeless in stretched cotton?
Nothing like a gentle reminder of what could have been if
they hadn't learned to say "no thanks, I'd better not".)*

"I think he may be a bit too bright for me though, always
one step ahead while I'm still putting my daps on. He
told me someone he knew had a stroke, right? And the
only things he could say were tea, no and fuck off. Turns
out he was having me on. So I told him I could speak
three languages just to get back at him – but I didn't tell
him they're English, Bullshit and Obscene. He did tell
me he likes exercising and goes jogging every night. I
know that's true because he's got dirty trainers in his
porch and a kagool. I mean what gay man do you know
who would be seen dead in a kagool unless they were
going out running?"

*(I used to run. I got up to a few miles on the treadmill
once upon a lardy time or two. God, I felt invincible then.
Really fit, almost normal, but utterly proud of myself. I
wonder where that pride went? Did I eat it?)*

"So I noticed then that I was holding my stomach in
when he was talking to me. Well, I didn't want him to
see my belly did I? Do you think he'll think I'm fat,
Han? Should I take up exercising? Do you think he'll go
off me because I've got a belly? Han! Do you think it'll
put him off? Can you get big knickers for men? Should I

look for a pair. Stupid. You're just being stupid… what if he likes fit men? I'm not fit, am I? But I'm thin. Do you think it'll matter? I really like him too. He says he's got really crunchy Altoids… I mean deltoids! I think I need to go on a diet."

(Diet. Die-yet. Crunchie. Oh Christ…)

> ## It's not whether you get knocked down; it's whether you get up
>
> ### Vince Lombardi

I'M GETTING FED UP with writing this column. Sorry! But I've said it now.

Not because it's a chore, but because all I do is moan about what I've NOT achieved.

I haven't exercised for weeks, haven't seen personal trainer Abs for ages (my fault, or rather the fault of increased hours in work), and I'm as defeatist about it all as per usual.

And still, bless him, he keeps in touch with tips, words of encouragement and e-mails to get me going. Poor dab – I told him I'd be a challenge, but I bet he feels it's like climbing a mountain of frustration wearing nothing more than a scowl.

But there is some good news – I lost EIGHT POUNDS last week.

And no, it didn't fall out of my purse. Even so, a sneaky sideways glance at myself in the mirror led me to assume it's gone off my eyelashes.

So I've done that desperate of desperate things and gone back on the Atkins diet.

I lost a couple of stone on it before, about three I think.

But it was an absolutely miserable time for me.

If you're a big meat eater, it's fine but, sadly, I'm not. And as I don't like a large variety of food anyway, even when not watching my calories, it's hellish.

But it gets the weight off without worrying about going to the gym.

The docs are split on its virtues though.

One I met told me it was the embodiment of calorific torture; another said, and I quote, "Bugger what other people say! You look fab and you're losing weight – and that's the most important thing in the long run."

So, as ever, those around me who love me and want me to flourish have gone out of their way to fill up my cupboards with trays of eggs, packs of ham, enough chicken to last a lifetime and door stop-sized pieces of cheese.

And that's about it – eggs, cheese, bacon and ham. That's my staple diet now.

Breakfast is impossible as you'd have to fry bacon, and who has the time?

Atkins isn't a cheap or quick way of losing weight, but it's always worked for me.

It's one of those diets where you don't have to moderate your intake – and let's face it, we chronic (in more ways than one…) dieters are useless at moderation.

Basically you can eat what you like – you're just not allowed to make a sandwich out of it.

A little bit of what you fancy? You might as well be talking gibberish to me.

I won't stay on it for long, just long enough to get to the point (in my mind at least) where my cheeks don't crush my fringe when I smile.

So that's where I am this week – eight pounds lighter, growing feathers and still unfit.

I hate the idea, if I'm perfectly honest, of going back to the gym once my working pattern reverts to something near normality.

I hate it – but as someone close to me said the other

day, do I hate the way I am more? I'm tossing a coin as we speak. Hey, at least it's not a stack of pancakes, right?

It's OK to be fat. So you're fat. Just be fat and shut up about it

Roseanne Barr

IS IT POSSIBLE FOR your trousers to get tighter overnight?

Or is it, like most things to do with me, simply in my head?

I swear to you that sitting on the train yesterday morning, I felt my belly had expanded so much over the weekend it was nudging the bloke in front of me.

Things continue to go awry – this has been a mixture of being given new responsibilities at work, thereby not being able to meet trainer Abs at allotted times; Abs being on a course (but those kind souls at the Lifestyle Palace did call me up and give me the option of seeing someone else); and me being generally, well, me.

And yet, last week, something happened to me, some little change to my routine, which has taken me away from thinking about my body, to thinking about the health of my heart.

It's amazing that when you have something else to think about, apart from yourself and your perfect imperfections, you start to feel healthier in general. Or at least I do.

Food has been almost a secondary thought and that's a full fork-tongued curse because:

1 – I don't eat enough
2 – I forget to eat
3 – When I do eat, and because I'm feeling happier, I

eat my own body weight in cheese on toast before I realise what I'm doing.

But at least, for the moment, it's being done with a big smile on my face.

I miss Abs, though. I miss his gentle persuasion, his wise words, his washboard belly and Scottish tones.

I don't want to go with anyone else, because in fitness and health terms he has my heart. I'm just sorry that the way to it is through my belly and being allowed to slump on the settee, thinking defeatist thoughts.

The next time I see Abs, he's going to measure me. This, he says, is to judge my progress and get me away from thinking about my weight in terms of boulder-sized stones and changeless pounds.

And I'm fine with that, with the measuring, and talking, and trying not to eat bread while I'm waiting for my tea to cook.

It's just that this all tends to smack of the fitness equivalent of spending hours preparing my files before actually revising for my A-levels.

I convinced myself that the preparatory work was the REAL work, that it HAD to be done, when all I was really doing was putting off the inevitable.

And that was pushing myself out of my comfort zone and trying to be, as someone dear to me said this week, working towards being the best Hannah Jones I can be.

I just wish I knew where to start.

I burned sixty calories. That should take care of a peanut I had in 1962

Rita Rudner

GUESS WHAT, I'M GOING swimming tonight. Can you imagine what's going through my mind right now?

Not only do I have to content myself with the worry of stripping off in front of others – last week I was recognised in the changing rooms while pulling off my work knickers! – I'm coming out in a nervous rash thinking about walking into the pool area, getting INTO the pool, swimming like a lead weight, men seeing my underwater fat 'bits' through their goggles, getting OUT of the water, drying in front of strangers, and getting changed.

I've got to shake my head in wonder when people say to me, "Why don't you go for a walk? How about a swim? Hey, fancy a bike ride?"

What these well-meaning souls don't realise is that the nonsense that surrounds activity is far worse than the hard work involved in actually doing something active.

Abs, my Scottish saviour, totally gets this, though – or so he says.

Although he doesn't quite understand my vanity (I'd swap that word for nervousness or frustration), he knows a commitment to fitness and diet is much bigger than I am – and I AM a big bugger.

He knows, for example, that I like boxing – so that's what we do during our hour together.

He also knows I hate talking about diets – so he sets out some easy challenges for me and tries to talk sense AT me while I battle with doubts and divisions ("walk upstairs to get some water Hannah and go downstairs to go to the toilet, and keep some grapes on your desk and you don't eat enough"). He knows I feel utter unease walking into that gym – so he starts talking to me about something else and suddenly I realise I'm on a treadmill and I've been walking for 10 minutes. UP HILL.

He stretches me, philosophises at me, coaxes me, talks at me, pulls at my laziness until I can feel my muscles loosen. But more than that, he absolutely makes me feel capable of getting fitter.

I don't think he hears my silent frustration as he instructs me how to slide up and down a mirrored wall with only a giant ping-pong ball for support.

But I imagine he can see the hope in my eyes, and less of the honey-coated glaze.

So what if it's clouded by years of self-doubt, inactivity and layers of lard?

It's there, easing me back into a body image reality which hasn't been distorted by years of indifference.

But asking me to take off my clothes and start on the first of the 40 lengths he's asked me to swim this week?

Seems like asking me to put my heart on a plate and kick it into touch.

But I'm going to go for it. There'll just be more water falling from my eyes into that heated blue oasis of my potential as I go.

> **Aidan: Well, if Miranda doesn't want the kid, can't she just give it to Charlotte?**
> **Carrie: No... it's not like a sweater**
>
> *Sex And The City*

SOMETHING IS GOING TO happen at about midday today which has made me stop and think about my well-being.

It's about then that my mother will call me to tell me the sex of the latest member of our already tiny family.

My auntie, 41 now and a life-long kiddie avoider if I'm honest, is having what the Yanks call a C Section this morning.

And with it comes the threat that 'the thing' will be given to me for holidays while its ma and pa go on theirs together, and also if anything happens to either one of them.

Let's get this straight now – I'm not really maternal, neither do I shy away from kids.

Give me one with a cheeky face, fat cheeks, dirty knees and who knows how to be entertaining and full of personality without being a precocious nightmare, and I melt.

But the idea of being totally responsible for one? It's bigger than me – Jesus, it's even bigger than my belly and that has its own postcode.

I've been unable to see trainer Abs because of work commitments, but he's sent me a list of things I need to do while we're estranged. I read them – a veritable smorgasbord of challenges to pick at, which I promptly

28

put in my To Do From Monday list.

If I could come to terms with how I look, without that shaky self-perception that makes me uncomfortably, well, *Me* at times, I'd say bugger it to this diet and exercise lark and start on a different kind of journey – and that would be to have a love-in with myself and say, hand on heart, Han, you're not all that bad, you know.

But with another little life about to enter mine today who will need me to be around for a long time, maybe this will give me the final push I need to be better and fitter and healthier than I am.

And it's been a good morning so far – no cigarettes, no butter on my toast and no sugar in my tea, all in the name of keeping 'clean' and healthy for baby.

But the thought of maybe bringing up said baby without such treats for the rest of my life?

I'm too much of a Big Baby to contemplate it.

> **You have to stay in shape. My grandmother, she started walking five miles a day when she was 60. She's 97 today and we don't know where the hell she is**
>
> **Ellen Degeneres**

IT'S BEEN A BAD week. It all kicked off when trainer Abs had to cancel our sweat fest at the gym.

And yes, sadly, I am being clean.

Via text, we arranged to meet the next day only for me to wake up feeling sapped of energy in the build-up to the Curse Of Eve week.

Girls, you know where I'm coming from, right?

Combine that with a hellish week at work and this blasted anaemia, which the bright sparks are failing to plug with three pills a day, and the last thing I wanted to do was exercise or watch my food.

A week later, it's still rumbling on and I'm feeling that old nudge of defeatism jabbing at me again.

Abs can't do this week either, so I'm left with some big dilemmas about doing this on my own.

And frankly, I don't trust myself to love myself enough lately.

OK, so that may sound a bit too much Oprah and less Welsh than I'd like, but anyone who's loved and not lost in the diet game will know what I'm on about.

On the plus side – and trust me when I say I'm rummaging through the empty pizza boxes of my mind to find something positive to say about the last seven days –

I have done a few lengthy walks with the dog.

I didn't go swimming again, but I persuaded myself I was taking a step in the right direction when I got myself a new swimming costume.

It's black, it comes with its own scaffolding system for my belly and boobs, and yet, curiously, it's also fitted with a zip just in case I fancy showing off a bit of cleavage.

The last time I was in the pool, this girl paraded around like she was on a beach in Ibiza.

I mean, who puts on a white bikini just to swim one length and then walk, arms over her head like she's saluting the sun (and obviously giving herself a nicer line in Svelte), playing with her hair like she's being filmed as a Bo Derek stand-in?

Umm, not me. I was too worried about said scaffolding, walking to the dressing room without slipping, and trying to get undressed under a flannel-sized towel so that nobody else – especially Bo – could see my bits.

But there is hope. I think. Abs is back on Friday – and I can only pray my enthusiasm returns with him

> **Reality check: you can never, ever, use weight loss to solve problems that are not related to your weight. At your goal weight or not, you still have to live with yourself and deal with your problems. You will still have the same husband, the same job, the same kids, and the same life. Losing weight is not a cure for life**
>
> **Phillip C. McGraw**

A FEW THINGS HAVE happened to me since I last wrote.

I, and don't ask me how, lost more weight – a few pounds off my cuticles and counting now. I can't see it going from any other place on my body.

I'm back doing my 'normal' job so I'm able to start back at the gym with Abs today (set your watches for 4p.m. as I set myself a mission not to shout in frustration at myself via him).

Someone close to me disappointed me so right on schedule, I reached for 20 fags, a can of full-fat Coke, a big packet of big crisps and a giant bar of Fruit & Nut while trying to make sense of it.

(Note to self: try Galaxy next time, it lasts longer when you suck it and drips less when used as a biscuit replacement in tea.)

There isn't a number four thing that happened to me, but I'm trying to exercise my fingers to make up for the fact I've not bothered with the rest of my body for the past six weeks.

Abs suggested something to me last week which

caught me a bit on the hop.

He asked if I'd considered actually paying for some extra sessions, as I get my membership at the Lifestyle Palace and hourly session with the great man gratis.

To be honest with you, I hadn't given this any thought at all, prior to his suggesting it.

I mean, you, me, him and the wider world all know how useless I am when left to my own devices.

Why hadn't it occurred to me that I could actually put my money where my (usually full) mouth is and see him for another shorter session? I'm tight and stupid, obviously! So I'm juggling my finances about, seeing if I can afford it.

My mother, of course, would have no hesitation in saying I could.

"Give up the fags and take sandwiches to work – you'll save a fortune," is her wise and sensible advice.

My timely response would be, "But Mam, I like my fags and I'd only eat my sandwiches by the time the train got to Caerphilly anyway!"

I know what I'm like, she knows what I should be like, and I try to operate somewhere between the two poles.

Carbs shouldn't come into the equation (I'm off the Atkins by the way) and neither should that shaky conundrum of my self-worth being rooted in the size of my waist or reflected in the treatment of me by other people.

Life's often shit – but at least I'm toying with the idea of paying out a little extra each week to ensure mine's less of one in the long term.

There are two kinds of people in the world: those who love chocolate, and communists

Leslie Moak Murray

SHIT, I CAN'T CRACK the food thing. I find jogging easier, and I can't do that without coming out in hives and arranging a bionic transplant to remove my boobs, putting cold compresses on my black eyes to bring the swelling down and arranging new legs and lungs.

While I was punching personal guru Abs in a boxing session last week, he talked at me about eating more regularly. And I couldn't help but sound defeatist as the poor bugger tried to console me.

"Have fruit in your porridge," he suggested.

"I don't like fruit," was my reply from the baby walker.

"Eat fish at least three times a week then," was another stab in the dark.

"Ummmm, I've got this fish phobia, see. And if someone else is eating it I have to leave the room."

"How about turkey? Salad? Jacket spud? Keeping grapes on your desk?"

"Oh dear... no. Sorry. Ummm... maybe I'll try the grapes thing. Can they be seedless though?"

You see my problem? It's not that I'm trying to be difficult, I just don't like even an average variety of food.

My trouble is that I eat too much (but apparently not regularly enough) of the little I do like.

I did do the grapes thing though.

But being a foodie, someone who doesn't think of

34

food when they're eating (just every other waking moment), I ate four pounds of grapes before I'd even realised I was playing catch with them in my mouth, like some cheap Z-lister circus act with no (Billy) Smarts to speak of.

The good news is that I went swimming twice last week, and did ten more lengths than Abs had asked me to do – 50 – breaking my personal best (and nearly my back in the process). Then again, my previous personal best was three in 1977.

I've walked the dog, taken the stairs instead of the lift, did a bit of stretching and have even frozen the bread in my house so that I'm not tempted to nibble while I cook.

And hey, I was the little kid who used to eat frozen Arctic Rolls every Sunday as I couldn't wait for them to defrost!

I'm not above such behaviour now, if I'm honest.

But I am above, I hope, not doing something about it in the morning.

> # I mean, I never had an image of myself as a fat person. While I knew I was fat, I didn't see myself that way
>
> **Doyle Brunson**

I ONCE BOUGHT A car wearing a towelling bath robe.

May I just add that it was a bleach-soaked bathrobe to boot.

There I was, chewing the fat about advertising and what-not with one of South Wales's biggest car dealers – I was editor of the Gwent Gazette at the time and trying to sound important, granted – when I suddenly noticed my coat had pockets.

Oh, there's odd, I recall thinking. How come I hadn't noticed those before even though I'd looked for them?

Of course, my proper coat didn't have pockets and still doesn't – the bathrobe, however, did. Two of them. Ripped. Hanging off. Literally by four threads.

So I rushed over to talk to my father, in a panic about looking stupid while trying to sound not so, and the conversation went like this.

Me: "Dad, I'm wearing my bathrobe! It's covered in bleach as well!"

Dad: "I know. I saw you leave the house wearing it."

Me (confused): "You saw me leaving the house with it on and you didn't tell me?! Why?"

Dad (straight-faced): "Well, I thought it was all the rage now."

Typical. Anyway, this all goes to show how easily I fall from my own sense of grace. As soon as I FELT silly, I started to have fat thoughts.

I slide with ease into these negative associations, unlike the times I tried to get down actual slides without the use of a vat of Vaseline and an industrial-sized hoist. When I was a kid I avoided the predicament by having my own playground at the back of The Castle, my family's pub, to be shielded from any kind of embarrassment.

I can laugh about it now, of course, chuckle at the day I bought a car wearing a bathrobe and how easily I raced from confident to cry baby, thinking that all anyone would ever really see was the size of the joke, and not the girth of me or the circumference of the bleach splatters (to say nothing of my arse).

I got to thinking about this after reading the answers to questions I had set the cast of an S4C comedy about a car dealership for a feature I was doing.

But I have to say neither mine nor their driving stories were as funny as my lodger Hiya Love's, the fount of all mishaps and mayhem, the only person I know who'll wash windows when the Jehovah's Witnesses are going past so he'll be assured of someone to speak to.

On his driving test 'down the country' – as we Ebbw Vale natives call anywhere north of Brynmawr – the instructor turned to him on his test, four weeks after his 17th birthday, and said, "Very good, Mr Amphlett. You've done really well. All that is left now is a few questions on the Highway Code."

"Can you please tell me why you should always wear sensible shoes when driving?"

"Well, you don't know who you're going to see in Abergavenny on market day," says Jon, in all seriousness.

Composing himself after acknowledging his fuzzy

37

logic, Mr Instructor then asked, "And can you name me a sign you're more likely to see here in the country rather than in a built-up area?"

The answer was iconic, "Pick your own strawberries."

Oh, strawberry jam and crumpets… Sorry, where was I?

> ## Anyone who uses the phrase 'easy as taking candy from a baby' has never tried taking candy from a baby
>
> ### Anonymous

I'VE BEEN ON HOLIDAY.

Well, not holiday in the sunning yourself (ugh… not for this November baby) and relaxing sense, but one where I was stuck indoors with a screaming newborn who thought my fluffy jumper and even fluffier bathrobe were decidedly womb-like.

I kid you not when I tell you that said baby became cooing sweetness personified when in my arms, a curious thing really, as I'm hardly maternal. But his mother, a first-timer at 41, was glad of the break and, as such, thanked me in the only way she knows how – in the currency of carbs.

Baby's mother, who is the same size in clothes as she is in her tiny-toed shoes, used to call me a 'fairy camel' when I was (not so) little, and would run screaming to her mother – my nan – that I was eating chocolate gateau (ALL of it, and still while frozen… well, it saves dirtying spoons, was my odd-bod thinking).

And she's blamed my family's enjoyment in watching me eat and their inability to say no to me, for my weight 'problem' ever since, so there's a nice, neat, little connection for you.

How did I get so zaftig-like and, here's a thing, nurturing? It wasn't by eating a banana for breakfast and yoghurt for lunch, I can tell you.

Anyway, their portion sizes are normally enough to feed an anorexic Munchkin – I'm talking five spuds between five and a scoop (and I mean ONE scoop) of ice-cream for afters here – but as I was doing the cooking (grilled, as ever; fat-free, always) the portion sizes increased accordingly to what I would deem as 'normal'.

But because I was stuck in the house with nothing to do, bar look doe-eyed at the baby in my arms and feel the kind of connection with him that I'd only previously read about, what do you think I did?

No, not take the baby for a walk, or dust.

I ate. Fresh bread. Full-fat butter. Strawberry jam. Sugar in my tea. Toast. Hobnobs.

I filled up on nonsense as it was there, I was bored in between feeds and I used that old deceiving device of reminding myself, "Han, a little of what you fancy on holiday is fine, everyone does it."

I forgot to remind myself that baby boot camp in Skipton hardly qualifies for self-indulgence à la fortnight in Venice.

But just think of the damage I would have done with pizza…

> **I have always wanted a mistress who was fat, and I have never found one. To make a fool of me, they are always pregnant**
>
> **Paul Gauguin**

I HATE WEARING A bra. When I go home after work, the first thing I take off is the old twanger.

If I could get away with doing it on the train, I would – but who wants black eyes? Or people staring at the sad pair of spaniel's ears otherwise known as my boobs.

I am what's known in the industry as a big girl. So walking into a 'normal' shop to buy a pretty over-shoulder boulder-holder has never been an option for me.

Instead, it's always been off to Evans playing the game of 'Guess My Size' or sending off for some monstrosity from a free catalogue.

And EVERY single one I've ever owned has stuck in me, the one underwire (always just the one) drops out, it's been too tight/high up at the back, made me droop, made me uncomfortable, gave me the support of a wet lettuce in a piece of cotton and felt like if I raised my arms over my head my legs would follow in sympathy.

I went to Evans a while back and got measured, the lady there coming out with a curious mixture of numbers and letters that were off the Richter scale.

Thinking they had it wrong, I trotted off to M&S and the fitter there was very helpful, if a little condescending when it came to the body shaper I was wearing (or, rather, my body shape).

She said they would find a bra "even big enough for

41

you, love" and they did – two 44DD examples of semi-torture.

Of course, as soon as I put them on I was immediately lifted (both boobs and spirit, if you know what I mean), but after two hours of wear I felt constricted and restricted.

So when it came to getting measured in Leia, I was a little sceptical.

I'd seen the flimsy, sexy numbers in the window (ah, a girl can dream can't she?) but didn't think they'd be able to find one to fit me.

But they did. And, like a big-boobed Victor Kiam, I was so pleased I bought the company (well, not really, but I did buy a company-endorsed black bra for £32).

After hearing those shock words – "Yeah, just as I thought, you're a 42G" – I started to get depressed about the choices available to me and the sheer SIZE of my fried eggs with hats on – they still don't look THAT big, do they?

Would my literally ample bosom mean the only bras available for me would be chewing gum white bolsters, the kind which look like sling shots for cannon balls when on the line?

Surprisingly the choice was really good, and I came out of the shop with a beautiful black bra and a skin coloured one.

Thinking about it, and although my Leia size still hasn't sunk in, I'm more comfortable in my new size bra than any other one I've had. Honest! It doesn't jut out like spiked wings at the sides, the wire doesn't stick in me, the cups fit closely to my skin – on the downside, the straps do feel a little tight, though.

But my new bras do have that all important component that's normally missing in us big gals' wardrobes – it's really, really pretty. Sadly, I think it loses its lustre on me. Because you've got to feel sexy before you stand a chance of looking sexy, right? And this is where things start to droop for me, in more ways than one.

RIGHT, IT'S TIME. IT'S time to sort this out once and for all.

I've got two big dos coming up and the thought of going shopping for them is bringing me out in pre-performance tics.

There's more to this being big lark than meets the eye, you know.

Not only do you have to consider what you're going to wear and if your legs will chafe in it, you also have to accept that you are incredibly limited in what you can buy.

Someone I know spent a few hours surfing the web last week looking for 'outsize' smart clothing suitable for the Baftas and a wedding (my two dos).

And she – a sympathetic size 12 – said she was amazed by my lack of options.

Sadly, I'm predisposed to the option of not going at all and that's because I always feel, well, better-suited to being unbooted, stretched out on the settee in my comfies.

Although I can spruce up with the best of them, I'm mindful that I have to do that dance, when you're big, of drawing attention away from the flesh and taking it directly to the face.

Said in an Aussie-like Kath and Kim drawl, it's more

"look at moieeeeeeeeeeeee" and not "oi, ok, I know I've got a belly and big tits, but wouldn't you rather look into my eyes instead?"

So the depressing realisation that I needed to go clothes shopping has put me in a tailspin.

This morning I've had breakfast, arranged two sessions with Abs at the gym, and thought to myself I WILL change my life and habits this week.

At the BBC yesterday morning, a handsome high-flyer with shiny shoes told me my column is one of his favourites.

There we were, chewing the (my?) fat at 7am, talking about training and sweating and what-not, when he asked me how it was all going.

And I did that big girl thing where I played the self-deprecating card, pointed to my assembled body bits and said, cheeky grin firmly in place, "As you can see, handsome boy, it's going really well and my body is now a temple. Pass me a doughnut on your way past, will you?"

Ooooh, how we laughed – and ooooh, how I really felt like saying, "Actually, it's going as badly as it always does, with me oscillating between feeling like saying bugger it to this diet and exercise lark, and looking downcast at my inability to move my ample arse and do something positive to shrink it."

But at least I DID have breakfast this morning, I DID avoid the doughnut and Abs WILL be on my case in a double header this week.

And that's the best I can do – I mean, how's a girl expected to use free weights when she's got loads of worrying to do?

I'm good, but I ain't that good.

> # Fat people are brilliant in bed. If I'm sitting on top of you, who's going to argue?
>
> **Jo Brand**

IN THE WORDS OF stand-up Totie Fields, "I've been on a diet for two weeks and all I've lost is two weeks."

Adapted by me, "I've been on a diet for 52 weeks times 34 years and all I've lost is the ability to work out on the calculator how many weeks I've lost in total."

Honestly, I'm thinking of giving up dieting as a bad idea, telling the eternal ally and foe called Fatso Face Jones, "Yeah, I'm Fat. So?"

And then, after I imagine myself shouting this at a mirror while standing naked in a 'getting to know myself' pose (dear God alive...), I come out in a cold sweat thinking that I would die if anyone – ANYONE – called me the 'F' word.

See the conundrum?

If you're anything like me, when things are going OK you totter around like a mild-mannered diva, thinking that you've at least got something going on.

But as soon as a negative happens or a seemingly innocent comment is made about my looks, the diamonds nestled in my belly button suddenly turn into charcoal, dirtying up my once healthy mind with big, black smudges of doubt.

Once upon a time, I fancied this bloke. Looking back now, I've no idea why – he talked at me with his eyes half open and didn't have many teeth. He didn't bite, but

I imagine he'd give my phizog one hell of a suck.

Anyway, Dwayne Pipe, as I like to call him, didn't suffer from any lack of self-confidence, didn't notice he wasn't spending much time at the dentist's or that he needed to open his eyes more.

And I, for some bizarre and doubtlessly needy reason, was simply fascinated with him.

This one day, while out walking together during a university jaunt for a philosophy seminar, I felt so good about myself I was convinced there was a wind machine blowing my hair in lots of beautiful directions, that my make-up was flawless and that I looked fantastic.

I was getting attention, I was with someone who I thought was finally noticing me blah blah blah, so the upshot was I wasn't emotionally eating for comfort. I had it going ON!

Anyway, Dwayne Pipe turned to me, smiled a big toothless smile and said, in all seriousness, "Oh, Hannah, I think you're aesthetically very pleasing, really quite beautiful – it's just such a shame you're not into exercise or dietary control."

And that, shocked reader, is verbatim. It's OK to shut your mouth now.

The curious thing about this story is that I didn't crumble and self-negate at that moment – I remember flinging my head back and laughing like there was no tomorrow.

It was only later, when left to my own devices, that Dwayne's words stabbed me in the heart and I reached for the soothing embrace of 12 cheese and onion pasties. Luckily, I never reached for him again – because no man's worth snagging by making false promises of exercise or dietary control, however well intentioned.

Frankly, I'd rather be fat and have fabulous teeth than

be slim with my eyes half-closed to the wonder that is me.

Now where did I put my glasses?

> **Let me have men about me who are fat…**
> **Sleek-headed men, and such as sleep-a-nights.**
> **Yon Cassius has a lean and hungry look…**
> **Such men are dangerous**
>
> **Julius Caesar in Shakespeare's play**

I WAS NINE YEARS old, and so was he.

He played football, I played the Hammond organ.

His parents were teachers, one of mine owned a pub and the other made a living sailing around the world. He was close to his grandparents, we had an extended family so I lived with Nan and Grancha.

His dad drove a brand new blue Volvo whose dash seemed to me like a large, bright computer screen; Mam had a blue Avenger and you could only open the passenger side door with a screwdriver and a bit of oomph.

He said "Mum" while I shouted "Mam" and he had the longest eyelashes I had ever seen in my entire life.

He was thin and I was fat, but the details don't matter, nor does the fact that we had so little in common.

All the you need to know is that his name was Ian and he was my first real crush.

OK, so I'd had mini love-ins on the Fonz, Doyle from *The Professionals* and the blond one from *The Dukes of Hazzard.*

But Ian was someone I could cast furtive glances at during break time and he was the one I thought about every time I saw a blue Volvo go over the top road just above our pub, thinking that it was him coming to see

49

me.

But he didn't really notice me, as I was, as my father once playfully described, a bit of a pork pie – and that was Johnny Jones-speak for plump.

I wasn't a Julia (our school's real looker in skinny jeans) or Ruth (her equally sassy best friend in matching denim, so tight it made their legs look mistakenly as if they had rickets, in one school picture), but I was still in the 'in' crowd, even though said pork-pie status made me more of a pal than an object of age nine snogging desires.

But I still remember the day that Ian turned to me in Miss Morgan's class and said, "I like your new glasses, Han, and have you done something to your hair?"

I smiled, it seemed, for ever.

I've had a few crushes since – some of Duran Duran, David Sylvian and even Juliette Binoche (don't ask) – but I thought I'd grown out of them by the time I was in my early 20s.

I told myself I was too old to fancy blokes who were unobtainable, whose pictures I could cut out from a magazine and imagine doing unimaginables with.

But that was until someone told me to watch Top Gear.

Bored and with my latest thriller already read, I had nothing better to do than turn on the telly to see what all the fuss was about.

And there he was, Jeremy Clarkson.

From the moment I saw him, I knew I was back to being nine years old again, back to wondering if he drove a blue Volvo and if he'd like my glasses.

So there I was, at the grand old age of 31, with a sad crush on Mr Miserable.

I don't know what it is about him, but he has that unutterable phwoar factor that just allows me to reserve a row of first-class seats in my ridiculous flights of fancy.

In scene one, me and Crush are in a cab going to Pizza Hut and he's got enough pull to clear the whole place and book it just for us. And at the end of the all-you-can-eat buffet he licks MY fingers and goes, "I just love a woman with an appetite".

In scene two, I say thanks by turning up in the studio wearing just a dab of Sandalwood and a long mac (obviously with a swing to the back, as I don't do straight up and down or belted, even in dreamland).

In scene three, I'm introducing him to Mam and Dad and we're all amazed at his Dr Doolittle ability in calming down our psycho dogs Max and Bertie to whimpering masses of well-behaved fur.

In scene four, he turns up at my house in a Saab convertible and says there's a present in the garage for me.

And I walk in and there, covered in a giant-sized bow that you only see in the movies, is a soft-top blue Volvo (of course it doesn't matter to me that he gets a trade discount).

When I saw Jeremy – terrible name, but I forgive him – and developed my crush I discovered something new about myself too.

And that was the fact that for 20-odd years, I'd denied myself a fantasy life because I felt too bloated to enjoy one.

Since Ian and the Fonz and co, I had told myself that I was too old to have idle fascinations with the idle rich.

Since Clarkson came into my life, I've also learned that I'm an idiot. Because now I've realised that it's still OK to dream, to fantasise, to wonder, to think that maybe one day someone special will notice you – whoever they may be – and adore you just the way you are. Limitless love you know, one that's not limited by some cock-eyed notion of convention.

Fame doesn't come into it – feeling that you're good enough for your very own Mr Big does.

The thing is, you don't need to feel silly because you have a crush, be it on Jonathan Ross, your milkman or some Hollywood hottie.

Singer Justin Timberlake, for instance, thinks Oscar-winner Halle Berry is just the 'finest' woman in the world and Fred Durst from Limp Bizkit supposedly had it real bad for Britney Spears.

So, while Jeremy remains in my life only as a figure on the small screen and Ian is back in the pages of my youth, to the days when I pored over the pages of the Smash Hits annuals and told – yes TOLD – Simon Le Bon that he'd be better off living in Wales with me than touring the world, I've concluded that you're never too old or too good-looking or too rich or too ugly or too poor or too, anything, to fall in love, in like, in lust or into the loony bin.

Just don't forget to make room in there for two.

Or 22 – remember, you're the Queen in the kingdom of Crush.

And no bugger's going to say anything to you if all you want to do all day is eat cake.

> **Have patience with all things, but chiefly have patience with yourself. Do not lose courage in considering your own imperfections but instantly set about remedying them – every day begin the task anew**
>
> **St Francis de Sales**

SO, WHAT'S THE ONE thing I could talk for Wales about? Dieting and shaky self-perception of course.

So when the Beeb called me in the other day to masticate over these two things on the radio, I didn't exactly jump at the chance, but was sufficiently confident not to get that butterflies-on-acid feeling I normally have when I do a bit of broadcasting.

But for some reason, when Richard Evans started to ask me questions I became a mumbling, fumbling elephantine idiot with nothing to really say for herself apart from "yeah, I've been on diets – yeah, they've never worked for me. Ummm, that's it."

When he asked me why that was, all I could think of saying was "because I am useless" and when he wondered what diet I was doing now I simply said, "I'm trying to have breakfast today, Rich." As if that was enough.

That sentence alone speaks volumes, I think, for foodie types – but I don't think Mr E got that.

Besides, on the radio you can't see my face, the expression that says "well, duh!" that accompanies any comment about food, dieting and unsound self-perception.

For me, eating breakfast is a big deal – it's a diet must-do, a healthy lifestyle necessity I guess. And yet, it's a major challenge as it bores me. Not as much as the idea of peeling, then eating, fruit aggravates me, but it comes close.

But I think Mr E was expecting some big proclamation like, "Well, actually I'm thinking of knocking myself out with a cricket bat at meal times and sucking cabbage water through a straw as a dinner substitute. Failing that, I'm going to have my jaws wired, tie myself to a treadmill and see if they do head transplants on the NHS."

The thing is, for a compulsive over-eater and under-achiever (I meant in exercise terms, Mam) like myself, even a minor change like having breakfast is a massive turnaround.

The problem, however, is having the type of mind where all these little changes add up to something significant. In this area, I may have a leak.

Because what successful dieters have that can't be weighed, but can be measured over time is something I lack. Wait for it now… patience.

I don't have the necessary tools at my disposal to think that 15 minutes on the exercise bike today will add up to inch-loss six months down the line; that eating as low fat as possible for a few months will get me down to a size 20 which would open up a world of change for me.

See what I'm saying?

The 'one day at a time' philosophy is, for me, significantly outweighed by the pull of instant gratification and the jabbing realisation that change, enough change for me to see at any rate, is a world away.

When it could just be a bowl of bran flakes, eaten at

7.30am every day, away.

> **Sex keeps me in shape. I don't diet, I eat what I like. I love Mars Bars and I smoke and drink. But I love running off in the middle of the day to make love. It really burns up calories**
>
> **Lisa Snowdon**

HE TURNS TO ME on the roof of the coffee shop as I'm taking a bite of a berry blast muffin.

He smiles that beautiful beam of his, full of animation and crunched up wonder when he unwittingly turns into Samantha from *Bewitched*.

And he says, "I think you're lovely just the way you are. But, yeah, of course I agree with you, it would be nice if you lost some weight. I care for you so I think about the health stuff too."

Stop there. Rewind. Read that over again. "I care for you so I think about the health stuff too."

The (fat-free) muffin thereafter went down in lumps, the (skimmed) iced latte failed to cool down the burning sensation rising up in my throat.

At that moment, previously having felt as happy as I get in my skin, I started to feel awkward, unsightly, ugly and as though knowing me – let alone being intimate with or caring for me – is one big exercise in making allowances for me.

It was one of those 'if only you were A and B instead of F, A and T' moments which seem to litter my life and which, before now, have had me running for the safety of being alone and not seen by anyone with a vested interest in my heart.

The sentence, well-meant and said with a comforting stroke over my arm (now feeling like two separate hams attached to my shoulders and wrists with crazy glue), killed me. Honestly, I was crushed. A throw-away comment, which was obviously anchored with assurances that I am lovely yada yada yada, didn't reach my ears in a healthy way. Instead it was infected with crushing self-doubt, which manifests itself in me as a painful silence.

It's at these times, where my sense of balance has been ripped out from under my size 7s (wide-fitting only, if Clarks are reading), that I become a deaf-mute.

Mute, because I can't form a sentence once my ears have translated even the sweetest comment into bile and deaf, because at this stage I no longer hear nice things.

I become impenetrable and ineffably sad. I'm no longer fun, upbeat or the Hannah whose company someone may want to bathe in. Because in my mind, all I heard was, "When I'm with you, all I see is trouble. And that's because you're fat. Get me the nearest size 14 now! Do I think you're fat? Come on, your favourite meal is seconds."

Odd, isn't it? And no, I can't make sense of it either.

The pain on hearing ANYTHING to do with my body shape, size, or portion choices is palpable. I don't see straight then – I certainly don't think straight – and all I seem to do well is close down a little and become embarrassed for whoever it is with that has to be seen with me. Again I'll say it – odd isn't it?

Shove me in work and give me a tight-as-a-vice deadline, no bother; ask me to take a flight on my own, piece of cake; drop me into an unfamiliar situation and expect me to flourish, watch on baby.

Say something – anything – about my size or my allure, make passing reference to it, make an innocent statement, though, and my responses will belie my intelligence. Every single time.

I become inarticulate and an emotional retard. It's unsightly, unseemly and odd. Notice a theme here?

For me, the size issue is utterly emotive and inextricably wrapped up in my self-esteem. When I'm feeling attractive, I'm capable, loving, quick-witted, generous and have a clear head.

My other head isn't as cheery, though.

Like some plus-sized Worzel Gummidge, I become a pale imitation of myself once a negative perception of myself assaults my senses. I'd like to change my head then, just pop the negative one in the cupboard to chill out and reach for a more rounded (absolutely NO pun intended) alternative.

She'd be open to suggestions, less defensive, capable of seeing herself in a normal mirror instead of looking in old ones rescued from a skip outside a now defunct three-ringed circus.

My new head would have the same intellectual capabilities as the old one, but it would come complete with in-built emotion deflectors which would spring into action as soon as I felt threatened by that 'I'd be fine, if only… ' mantra again.

Head number two would be sensible, stick at things, wouldn't mind doing a bit of exercise a few times a week and wouldn't tell its mouth to say "I've got a bad leg so that's why I'm getting the lift to the first floor" as an excuse to someone who'd spotted me, or tell said leg to do an impression of Long John Silver just for added believability.

Today, though, I'm left with myself, and stuck with

the same old battered belfry.

But it does come with a good heart – and just in case anyone is wondering, it's attached to a lazy, shapeless, dissatisfied body that also has a clean bill of health.

> **If I had been around when Rubens was painting, I would have been revered as a fabulous model. Kate Moss? Well, she would have been the paintbrush**
>
> **Dawn French**

I WONDER IF 'NORMAL' women compare themselves to me?

It's got me wondering, big style. I'm what's known in the trade as a people watcher, which simply means I'm nosey.

I can sit for hours staring at people from behind the safety of my dark glasses, making silent judgments on the way they look, hold themselves, the breadth of the smiles on their faces, or the lack thereof.

And of course, I compare myself with them every single time. But does it work the other way round?

When women see me – I'm not going to even pose the question about fellas as I'd only tie myself up in knots – do they wish they were more like me?

I can't imagine it for a nanosecond, but I'm told stranger things have happened at sea – largely by my father who was in the navy for 25 years and couldn't swim a stroke. (His theory is that if you're in the water in the middle of the Atlantic, it's not really going to help you much. Guess he has a point.)

I can't help but play the compare and contrast game. I could play it for Wales, and then move on to do it at Olympic level.

So when I see someone slim(ish) – she's always

slim(ish), always in shoes I could only dream of wearing, always smiling, normally chopsing into a mobile phone, never sweating in this bloody heat we're having at the mo – I start to judge my allure by a set of simple criteria.

At the top is that little thought as to whether my imagined emotional and physical opposite is truly, positively, absolutely, look-at-me-fellas comfy in her own skin.

Because I'm convinced I don't. I don't know what it is about women who look at ease with themselves, or what sets them apart from me.

Maybe it's the simple fact that their legs don't rub together, their bras don't feel like they're garments of absolute torture, they don't have to walk while making sure their tops don't stick to their bellies (it's an art – write in for tips, girls), and they can wear a dress without sleeves and a cardi.

But what do they see when they look at me? And what impression would they have after having a conversation with yours truly?

I don't know. And not knowing is a cruel twist in my sobriety (thank you Tanita Tikaram).

In my saner moments, I'd like to think they would find me affable, possibly charming, the fast side of quick-witted, big-haired, smoky-eyed, tallish and sing-songy.

Perhaps I come across as someone happy to be who she is, someone without hang-ups (hello?!), content to swoon around in that proud way that not bad looking big girls who don't give a damn do.

Yesterday I walked into work with someone who is the size of my left leg. She looked lovely in big dark glasses, white skinny-legged trousers under a polka-dot dress. It was blazing hot – and I had a mac on (don't ask).

My shoes hurt (they're flat as pancakes), my bra felt like I had borrowed it off a Sindy doll, my belly was stretching against my trousers and screaming "let me the hell out, will ya?" and my top looked as if it had shrunk in the wash.

Yep, just a regular day at the office.

So skinny, lovely pal and I walked past some blokes and not one – count them – looked at me. I know, because I made it my life's work to look at them looking at us (or rather not US at all, but confirming my suspicions that I wouldn't get a look in).

True to form they all visually pawed my London set, brilliant friend, musing on something that could never be.

And I thought to myself, as I was making chum giggle and pouring out the compliments about her outfit (I'm like that – dead honest and never short of nice words) if she ever – *ever* – looked at me and thought, "God, I wish I was more like you, Han."

Of course, I doubt I have any qualities she'd want and I'd bet money on there being not a single physical trait of mine she'd covet.

But still, maybe she's wondered what it's like to be me, grey clouds, saggy bits and all.

The trick here, of course, is to be careful what you wish for as the custard's not always thicker – unlike my legs – on the other side. Now and again, I'd kill for a quick taste though.

> **Some people are fat and some are thin. Some people have fair hair, some are ginger. So what? It's never stopped me getting men**
>
> **Alison Moyet**

> **I don't believe that if you're big it's an excuse to hide away**
>
> **Anna Scholz**

WHO DO YOU ADMIRE? Do the dinner party thing if you like. Imagine who you'd like to have round for pie and mash. Work this out, and you'll have a ready made answer when the big pile of chips are down.

When I was little I thought I was the love child of 'Little' Jimmy Osmond and Purdy, from *The New Avengers*.

I had a page-boy haircut and used to wear a battered Welsh hat – the string was broken so I went around singing 'Long Haired Lover From Liverpool' into the one end, pretending it was a microphone.

With the hair, the hat and a bit of a voice there was no convincing me that I wasn't the daughter of Jimbo and the Purdster – though the lack of any kung-fu moves, plummy accent and an interest in genealogy should have been evidence enough. But there you are.

I loved that pair as much as I adored my Elvis is King knickers and red wellies. So If I'd been asked at the age of five who I wanted to share my Salt'n'Shake with, these would have been up there.

This curious fascination continued until I was about eight, the year I came across Betty Rizzo.

There I was, still with the pudding-bowl hair 'cut', still humming ridiculous songs in my little blonde head, still refusing to wear jeans, sitting in Brynmawr cinema.

I was watching *Grease*, my first grown-up film, which seemed to embody everything I thought was cool about America – big beef-burgers oddly made out of ham, huge strawberry milk-shakes, fast cars, big hair and people who seemed to sing all the time.

Hey that was my life (if you substituted a Thunderbird for a dirty blue Hillman Avenger which you had to open from the inside with a screwdriver).

Not for me the sickly musings of Sandy or a desire to be a 'Beauty School Drop-Out' (but I did go around in a hair-net for a week after watching Frenchy's dream sequence and Tampax in my ears after my nan told me they were to keep the noise out).

No, I was smitten with Rizzo, the too-cool-for-school leader of the Pink Ladies, the tart with a heart who got to belt out 'There Are Worse Things I Could Do' and snog Kenickie in the deal.

She was naughty, she was daring, she was foxy, didn't give a damn and kind of taught me what 'lousy with virginity' meant after singing it during 'Look At Me I'm Sandra Dee'. (Me: "Mam, what's virginity?" Mam: "Ask your aunty Pauline, love." Pauline: "I'll tell you if you put that chip down.")

Stockard Channing was 33 when she played the teenage Rizzo and opened my eyes to the nature of bad boys, pencil skirts, and the colour pink.

She's 60ish now and she's always been on my wish list of party guests, maybe just because she could tell me how to rat my hair, whatever the hell that is.

I'd also ask Alison Moyet round. I was a massive fan of hers when I was in my late teens. She was a real role-model for me, a singer with a big voice and even bigger boobs – she was like the 80s answer to Beth Ditto, only she liked blokes and had better dress sense.

Dressed all in black, she oozed power and an assured sexuality – she looked like someone you wouldn't mess with in a dark alley and who would eat men between slices of door-stop-sized bread.

She sang like she looked, full-bodied and throaty, her low tones and high notes blowing anaemic imitators out of the water. And for the first time I thought to myself, "If she can do it, so can I". 'It' being becoming comfortable as I am.

I got to talk to her about being a 'big' popstar years later for an interview before she did a UK tour.

Standing an Amazonian 5ft 11ins and with acres of wonderful flesh, she is anything but a poster girl for petite pop stars.

In the 80s, when she burst onto the scene as the 21-year-old towering half of the electro-pop outfit Yazoo, she filled a much-needed void in the UK's perception of beauty.

Big beauty that is, although I'm loath to tag her with the same label that seems to dog Dawn French.

She's always described as big AND beautiful (as if attractiveness found in someone over a size 16 needs to be qualified).

Moyet is clearly an attractive woman. Full stop. But what makes her even more appealing is her apparent ease with herself – particularly with her own size. But things weren't always so rosy.

In typical forthright Moyet style, her Essex brogue

thickening when she's got a point to get across, she said to me one day, "I'm fat, so what?

"I can tell you something for nothing, I've never once lost a bloke because of it.

"I've lost sexual encounters because I've been neurotic about it, about being big when I wasn't so accepting of myself, but I've never been turned down by a man.

"My weight can go up and go down – by about four stone, I'd say.

"Some people are fat and some are thin. Some people have fair hair, some are ginger. So what? It's never stopped me getting men.

"But I have to say that I have been insecure about the way I looked, if men would fancy me.

"I mean, I came into the music world quite by accident and then, all of a sudden, from living in Essex and looking as if I was someone who could deal with criticism like water off a duck's back, I'd go up on stage to collect an award or something and some cruel cow would look me up and down and question what I had on.

"I realised very early on that people could be cruel, and now, because everything hurtful imaginable has been said to me, I don't give a damn.

"But before that I was at a point where I didn't find any comfort in myself, where I felt I was just some hideous gargoyle who had to hide herself away.

"But I could still get a bloke, if you know what I mean. And I know plenty of skinny birds who weren't half as lucky as me."

I'm sat here and her blood and tears voice is cutting through the nonsense in my mind right now, the one which is mentally tasting what we'd have for that dinner of dreams.

Designer Anna Scholz would dress us all for the occasion. She's another good looking big girl who I also got to talk to and learned to greatly admire because of her 'stuff it' attitude. She believes that if you're a size 16 or over, people are going to notice you anyway.

So why hide yourself away?

This simple philosophy from Anna, quite possibly Britain's most successful designer for women of size, makes her unique in the fashion world.

This means that if you are, say, a size 20 and you fancy something your size 10 friend has bought from her range, you'll be able to get it in your size too.

Of course, this doesn't mean that you will look good in it.

Hot pants on a zaftig *do* look more like an ill-fitting belt after all.

But Scholz, whose clothes are brimming with invention and dripping in glamour, doesn't dress women who lack a sense of style or are short of self-expression.

What she does is help women flaunt their allure, whatever their hip measurements.

"Anyone can wear my clothes of course," Anna, herself a bountiful size 24 who stands at an impressive 6ft, said to me.

"But they're for people who enjoy self-expression. They're not at all mumsy and frumpy.

"I hate that stuff. I mean, I go into M&S looking for a swimsuit and the really funky ones are only up to a size 16. It's so frustrating.

"Don't designers think that women who are bigger know how to dress? They can look as good as a size 12 in things."

Although famed as a designer for larger women – Dawn French, Roseanne Barr, Queen Latifah, Macy

Gray, and La Moyet all wear her clothes – she shies away from being labelled merely as a market leader in 'big' fashion.

"I don't really want to make a size statement," she explained to yours truly. "Everyone is different so why should one end of the market be deprived of something that the other has access to?

"You can wear our collection if you are big, small, young or old. It does not matter.

"The purpose of my garments is to allow a person to be whatever they are and feel comfortable and confident whether they are a size 12 or 24.

"I design what I think is a great collection first and foremost and then I make those garments available for big people. It's that simple."

One of her most famous clients, the comic Jo Brand, was dressed by Anna for the Bafta awards in London.

She was, however, styled by acid-tongued clothes-horses Trinny and Susannah for their show *What Not To Wear*.

Jo was transformed from Doc Martin romper-stomper to class act in a chocolate-coloured skirt and top and long velvet coat with leopard-print lining.

"She looked wonderful," recalls Anna. "She's been back a few times since and she really looked fabulous that night.

"That said, I would have put her in something else but Trinny and Susannah wanted a really classy look. I would have loved to have seen Jo in a lace bustier." And she isn't the only one.

Necessity, as the saying goes, is the mother of invention.

So when Anna found herself in her native Germany as a larger than life – literally – teenager, she decided to make her own clothes.

A stint as a model and a supportive family unit gave her the confidence she needed to accept herself as she was; comments from women of all shapes, ages and sizes on her own unique style led her to study fashion.

The two sides of the same fashion-savvy and confident girl eventually morphed their way into a designer who's a woman's woman, someone not afraid of her flesh or dressing it up, down or in glorious Technicolor.

Anna's luxury clothes are designed for maximum impact, for the woman who is confident enough to show her cleavage without flaunting it. She is unique and, because this is high fashion time, cash smart.

So if you can afford to dress in Anna Scholz you'll get a glamorous, versatile wardrobe oozing sophistication.

"These are luxury items as the fabric I use and other materials, such as Swarovski crystals, don't come cheap," she says.

"My theory is that you should go for maximum impact. I don't believe that if you're big it's an excuse to hide away. The clothes I make dress women beautifully.

"The current autumn/winter collection is very feminine with a touch of bohemian chic.

"I've used loads of luxurious cashmere and rich velvets with delicate detailing in lace, chiffon and intricate hand beading.

"I like purples, chocolates, bejewelled colours, clothes cut really well on the bias to give a woman shape but that don't cling too much."

In Anna's hands, every goddess can rewrite the 'fat fashion' rules.

She takes denim in a new direction with effective hand beading and sequin detailing. And her favourite, a shimmering fitted gold mac, has enough sex appeal to heat up any cold night.

From red carpet glamour to easy wear T-shirts, asymmetrical twin sets and slim-fitting cashmere sweaters, her collections are for people who like clothes. Oh, and who adore themselves into the bargain.

"There's nothing we women of size can't do or can't wear," says Anna. "But on second thoughts, maybe we should stay away from cropped tops and hot pants!"

Thin people are beautiful, but fat people are adorable

Jackie Gleason

HERE'S A QUESTION I'VE been pondering lately and I admit to having rainbow- coloured reasoning about it.

Do I think I'm any less appealing, sexy, funny or – oops a daisy – worthy because I'm overweight?

In my odd little mind, I'd say yes – although I admit I don't feel it all the time – but I've absolutely no bloody idea where this type of thinking comes from.

I went to 'see' someone about it once, hoping that my new friend with some fancy certificates could shed some light on the Fun House mirror way I see myself.

And this wise woman, with all her years of studying the human mind, particularly of those people with weight 'issues', simply said to me, "Yep, your thinking's all to pot. You're like an inverted anorexic and you shouldn't trust the way you think about yourself. You need to relearn the rules."

Years before that, I'd gone to 'see' another certificated wonder who tried to reassure me of my worth by going, "Rest assured you're quite lovely – I refuse to treat people who are ugly anyway. They don't get through the door."

Honestly, that's what she said!

I didn't go round to her million pound house again, though – I don't fork out £25 an hour and not even get a cup of tea thrown in, to say nothing of talking over your problems while sharing a Chinese.

71

For me, self-acceptance is all about self-perception. It's just that mine has got cloudy.

I'm currently beating myself up because I want two pieces of toast – but NOTHING is just about having a piece of toast, is it? The conversation with myself over something so trivial is so complex, it's tiring.

So I ask myself if I would be able to stop at two pieces.

Wouldn't it be better if I had just one?

Hey, what if I put two slices on one plate, some cheese on toast on a second plate, would people in the canteen think I was trying out for a balancing act at the local circus?

Would I dupe them, and myself, into believing the toast was for me and the cheesy delight for my slim and gorgeous friend downstairs?

This is typical thinking for foodies and people with a rickety view of themselves.

Everything is loaded, even without cheese on top.

I wish, though, that I had that blind, damn-it attitude, as summed up by comic fattie Rosie O'Donnell.

She said, "I see shows on anorexia, and women look in the mirror and think they are fat. I am kind of fat, and I look in the mirror and I don't think I'm as fat as I am.

"But I don't have self-loathing because of it."

Does that mean she wishes she were fatter, or doesn't care that she's fat because she thinks she's utterly fabulous the way she is anyway?

Hmmmm. It doesn't matter which is true, I think, because the outcome's the same – and that's one of blind self-acceptance and lack of leakage in the regular thinking stakes.

I'll take an order to go, please.

And today I think I'll forego the extra mozzarella.

> # There is no excellent beauty that hath not some strangeness in the proportion
>
> **Sir Francis Bacon**

SO I'M AT A colleague's desk and leafing through what can only be called, ahem, a lad's mag. On the front there are four big pictures of nice looking semi-dressed women in ridiculous poses.

There's been some kind of poll, voted by men, who have picked a woman for every occasion.

In the same way that I'd pick corned beef and vinegar sandwiches on a crusty baguette, salt'n'vinegar crisps and a can of shandy for a long journey, women have been picked for their suitability in various categories.

So to marry, the blokes have gone for Jennifer Aniston. For the perfect body, it's Keeley Hazell (who?) and they want to get trapped in a lift with Tera Patrick (again, who?).

The wildcard of this category is Dawn French who is labelled as being "a fat bird to cushion the blow if the lift plummeted."

Aw, blokes and fat jokes, don't you just love 'em?

Anyway, the woman that men want to get a bit fatter is Kate Moss, while newly slimmer former Pop Idol Michelle McManus is in the list too.

Morbid curiosity, do you think? I think they've just lumped the former 'lumper' in to demean her once again. Cruel buggers.

So, who do you think they want to see slimmer?

None other than Charlotte Church.

The writers of the magazine, who must surely all be perfect specimens of manhood, admit that it's "pushing it" to call Charl fat, but she could "do with a curve-accentuating diet".

Some bright spark even goes as far as saying "Some people think Charlotte is big boned, but when was the last time you saw a fat skeleton?"

I can, however, tell you the last time I saw an insensitive man.

Now a couple of things happened when I was leafing through this pile of tat. The first was that a female colleague came over and said she was rattled by the nudity in the magazine, that on some 'deeper level' she tore herself up wondering if she'd feel sexier if she looked like the models.

So there she was, taller than me (and I'm 5ft 8in in my bare feet), blonder than me, a body lift slimmer than me (a size 12 maybe?), with ram-rod posture and a flat belly.

And there I was, sweating in this silly heat, wearing a dress undone over trousers, posturing for some TLC, a size 24 (ssssh...), a sun hating miserable cow, and all I can do is laugh.

Because for all our differences – and let's face it, she'd be more likely to appear in such a magazine than I would – I've never, ever, for one sticky moment, judged myself against such girls.

For one, large sums of money would need to be handed over for me even to stand, head cocked, with my finger in my mouth – I only do that after dipping it in lodger Hiya Love's bolognese sauce.

My colleague said she gets "really, really" annoyed by such magazines; again, we couldn't be more different. I just laugh at them and have a good old nose.

I'm not offended, I'm not judgmental. The only big ache I have is that I think, built like I am, I'd look absolutely ridiculous in nice lingerie or snapped doing a seductive pose.

In this aspect, I feel slightly short-changed on my notion of womanliness.

But I'm a long way from thinking that ALL men would look at me and scowl just because they wouldn't be able to take a picture of me contorting like some circus freak while contemplating eating a banana (think about it… and relax) and wearing not much lace.

You get my drift, right? The second thing to hit me was the way in which most people – and I'm logging most women in here as well as the majority of men – think that being over a size 12 means they are fat. HELLO? What planet are you on?

What does it say about the world and our wonky thinking when someone over a size 12 thinks that they're fat and, by cruel association, may take it to mean that they're also not worthy of being taken seriously?

Hey, I think it about myself but I can pinch more than an inch and I've had a lifetime of musing on my shortcomings as first a 'puppy fat' kid, then a big teenager, an overweight adult and now (look away, Mam) a 'clinically obese' adult.

So I know what it's like to judge myself against the natural average – scratch that, I know what it's like to judge myself against myself and my own set of high standards. But saying a size 12-plus is a porker? A 'fuller-figure'?

Please! I am not talking a size 14-16 or 'roly-poly' 18-20. But I am talking without the aid of my celebritese goggles, which zone in on the international language of euphemism.

I'm flummoxed by the current coverage of so-called 'curvy and voluptuous' stars like Charlotte.

On the one hand we're told that looking super-skinny is now deemed bad by the media, so why do magazines think simply adding the word 'curvy' to a picture caption will make it seem as if they're genuinely featuring fuller-figured celebrities on their pages? Let's look at the evidence again.

Catherine Zeta-Jones has great boobs and Beyoncé and Jennifer Lopez are known for their 'big' bottoms. But the last time I looked out over my fringe of reality, they still owned itsy-bitsy sized derrieres.

I for one am pleased to see skeletal celebs chastised, but claiming normal-sized women like Charlotte have a weight problem just because they go from a size 10 to a 12 is not an improvement.

We'll leave the last word on the subject to our 'curvy', Chinese food-loving, bacon sarnie-munching, Cheeky Vimto-swigging Crazy Chick. As she simply puts it, "I'm happy with my figure."

And so she should be – she's a perfect size 12, the lucky bitch.

> **I found there was only one way to look thin, hang out with fat people**
>
> **Rodney Dangerfield**

SOME PEOPLE TELL ME I'm stylish.

Don't laugh, it's true! Not that I'd ever make the list of one of the most stylish women in Wales – perish the thought that there'd be a fattie on there.

I, of course, think I always look like a sack of shit gone wrong. But we all know I'm not the best suited person to make judgements about myself.

So what makes me stylish (and, trust me, I am cowering when using the word, and wondering, when people say it, do they mean I'm stylish for a 'big girl' or if I'm stylish, full stop?).

And do I have any tips to pass on to would-be big-bellied goddesses who are struggling to find their own sense of style? God forgive me, but here's Jones' Drones on life after a size 14...

Get Big Hair

As American biggie actress Delta Burke said, "I like having big hair because it brings me closer to God." Never, *ever* leave the house without first back-combing your hair and stamping on your straighteners. Girls, if you've got loads of skin you don't want to do thin upstairs. Understand? 'Flat' should only be used to describe a dwelling on one floor. And if you're NOT a natural blonde, leave the peroxide alone – you'll only end up looking like a bland wannabe thinnie.

Go natural, but go big; don't do colour tipping, crimping, put clips in or wear bands. Watch *The Vicar of Dibley* if you want a laugh – don't look in the mirror.

Get Fitted

Hiding yourself in dark, baggy clothes? Step away now! It's an urban myth that bigger women only look good in flowing garments made out of T-shirt material. I look like an advert for badly designed leisure wear in baggy clothes. Oddly, in fitted dresses and jackets and tops I actually look like I have some sense of body proportion. And if I can take the dart and flare-fitted plunge, you can too. Trust me, you won't bounce on the landing.

Dress To Impress

My favourite winter/summer/autumn look is springing head first into a dress. It always has to be fitted, it should come with a scooped neck, preferably with side splits so you can get a flash of colour from your trousers when you walk. Did you get that? Yep, that's right, I said trousers. There's nothing nicer than a knee-length dress worn over wide-legged – ALWAYS wide-legged – trousers. You'll look quirky and a little distinctive, something bigger girls can take to the bridge and revel in.

The Basque Country

Knickers and bras? I swap mine every time for an all in one body-shaper. With these little babies, you don't have to worry about your love handles sticking out and costing you an extra ticket on the bus. They hold you in and pull you up, and give you a nice bit of cleavage to boot. But here is a word of warning – learn to go to the toilet without undoing the poppers. Honestly, if you've got a belly and you're in a cubicle that barely takes your hips, let alone your bad mood, it's not worth the struggle to be all 'proper'. Pull it to the side and pray for a good aim.

Tum Tum Tum Tum Tum!

Not that I love my belly – with my small ankles and big stomach, I think I look like an egg on legs. Because I hate it so much, I'll do anything to disguise it, save wrapping myself up in bandages and calling myself Mummy Jones. As such, I wear tops that are about four inches below my waistline. I don't ever wear cropped tops, tops that sit just on my belly button, or tops that cling. A girl doesn't want to get arrested for indecency, does she? Opt for a long blouse, preferably in a dark and luscious colour, and never wear a belt. What's that about? Give yourself a waist by buying clothes which are long, lined and slightly fitted – you don't get one by tying your waist so tight your fat runs down to your knees.

To Spangle or to Dangle?

Plain clothes don't have to mean dull clothes. If you want to dress like a Christmas tree with bad roots, get yourself a gold tight top, team it up with one of those ridiculous bubble mini skirts and some snow boots. I guarantee you, you won't be a laughing stock. NOT! Avoid busy patterns, cheap fabrics and ANYTHING in the wrong size. Don't squeeze into a smaller size just because you're convinced you really are a size 16. The only thing I squeeze into is a booth in Pizza Hut, and you can guarantee I'll be wearing a comfortable size 24 on the way to the salad cart.

Sans Sleeves

If you have been hit over the head with a hammer and have it in your obviously damaged mind to let your bat wings fly free, make sure you do a bit of covering up. Go for a pashmina and when you think all the eyes of the world are on you and your fascinating tales from World Wonderful, let it just slip delicately around your shoulders and make a play of shrugging it up only to let it fall down again. And repeat as necessary.

To Boldly Go...

Be bold, girls. But beware, bold doesn't have to mean brash. If YOU are big or at least a few stones away from a shrinking violet, make sure your jewellery is big, your hair bigger, your heels chunky, your clothes flowy while being semi-fitted (trust me, it can be done!), your make-up dramatic and your décolletage perky. Oh, and don't forget your talcum powder. If you have to ask me what that's for, I don't think you've ever gone clothes shopping in July...

> **After all the trouble you go to, you get about as much actual 'food' out of eating an artichoke as you would from licking 30 or 40 postage stamps**
>
> **Miss Piggy**

11.05am

I'M DYING FOR A chicken roll. I can smell toast everywhere, writers eating their morning treats from the canteen, washed down with a frothy coffee.

But I'm trying to be good – so good in fact that this morning I got off the train a station early so I could walk the 10 minutes to work; so good, Hiya Love made me a packed lunch – two chicken rolls – so I wouldn't be tempted to go out and overeat, "just for a little treat, just this once".

You know, like a packet of lo-cal chocolate or an extra slice of bread.

Yeah, we're talking big sinning here. Not. He also packed them up and put them in HIS bag. We then went to the train together but he elected to sit in another carriage.

In short, he took my chicken rolls with him – so that I wouldn't eat them by the time we got to Ystrad Mynach, a couple of stops up. He didn't give them back to gutsy me when we got off either – he made sure I couldn't see him the other end because, like most people, he just doesn't have the heart to say no to me. So to get round my little predicament, he just hid.

With my chicken rolls.

Now, with the smell of toast wafting around me, and three pints of water down my throat in a feeble attempt to fill myself up, I desperately want a roll. Just the one (I think, I hope). But I can't have one because what would I then have for my dinner?

I also don't have them here, with me, whispering sweet nothings in my ear. God, the conundrum is huge. I might call him and ask, child like, if I can have one. But that's silly, right? I mean, I'm an adult. A grown-up who can make decisions about when to eat a chicken roll and how many to have in one sitting/walking/hiding round the corner, right?

Wrong.

I am useless when it comes to portion control. I'll only crack it when Nelson gets his eye back. I am worse, though, when it comes to thinking that I will be like this forever.

11.26am

It's 11.26 am. And I have it! Had it, more like. I called Hiya Love and he's plonked a roll – yes, just the one – on my desk. I felt happier knowing it was there, but because of a mix-up in the details of the rendezvous with the object of my affection, I was going down one set of stairs while he was coming up the other.

And while climbing down, I realised how antsy I was feeling.

I also bumped into a girl in knee-high boots and black jumper dress coming out of the loos playing with her hair, you know, in that kind of twiddly way that girls happy in their skin do to make us mere mortals want to punch them. Just the once you understand. Out one door and through another, and I'm assaulted by a woman shaped like Aphrodite – big boobs, little hips, loads going on – who's nibbling on a satsuma.

Yes, a satsuma.

And there I was, rushing because I want just the one roll, consumed by the consequences of this itsy-bitsy dilemma, wondering if I'll ever be a hair twiddler.

You know what I mean. I was disappointed in myself for giving in. A chicken roll, you see, is a metaphor for my dieting life – I'm obsessed with having it/not having it and all I can hear is the white noise in between the nonsense that accompanies free choice.

But I only have one life. Just the one.

(Unlike the roll, which tasted bloody lovely, so it consequently became two in my belly within 21 minutes of tasting the first.)

> **Instead of beating myself up for being fat, I think it's a miracle that I laugh every day and walk through my life with pride, because our culture is unrelenting when it comes to large people**
>
> **Camryn Manheim**

DO YOU EVER WONDER what other people's lives are like?

I do it all the time. I imagine what's on their walls, what's in their fridge, what the inside of their car looks like, where they do their shopping, if they eat dinner sitting at a table or balancing a tray on their lap.

Perhaps I'll go as far as musing on their brand of toothpaste, if they eat out much, or prefer to cwtch up with a loved one on the settee. I know it's silly and ridiculous, and all other kinds of grown-up adjectives you can throw at me, but I can't help but wonder how the other half lives and if it's as perfect as it sometimes appears.

So I was keen to interview Lucy Dahl and ask her about her childhood and if it was all that I imagined it to be.

True to form, her super dad, super author Roald Dahl, filled her, and her brother's and sisters' lives with laughter and mischief, mayhem and magic.

Hearing her talk about her inventive father's special take on mealtimes and bedtimes made me hark back to my own childhood.

Of course, my father wasn't an established author

(more like a tattooed old sea-dog) and he didn't read me stories he'd actually penned.

Instead he'd make my small corner of the world shine with tall tales of new furry friends.

Although there wasn't a Willy Wonka in sight, I had Harold Hare and Timmy the Tortoise and Old Farmer Giles.

Anyway, Dad Jones would combine my love of animals with my greater passion – Sunday dinner. Yep, he knew how to pique, then keep, my interest.

I remember going mad with desire thinking about these three getting together and sharing a Sunday dinner made with buckets (say it slowly now) of dark, rich, thick gravy – BUCKETS! – and Yorkshire puddings the size (hear my oooohs!) of a bungalow.

You may also imagine me, aged about five, putting my fingers over my ears and screaming "Stop it now mun Dad!" as he tantalised me with stories that made me smile second, salivate first.

He may not have been Roald Dahl, but he was my champion of the world. I mean Yorkshires the size of houses? No bloody contest.

But what damage did it really cause me, stories inexorably linked to what I could put in my mouth?

I never thought such stories, all linked to food, would have had any deep psychological impact until I met Janet, one of the most remarkably insightful thinnies I've ever had the good fortune to spill my half-baked, sugar-free beans to.

She was yet another 'professional', someone who, in a series of sessions where I struggled to string a sentence together about My Fat Life and lack of self-confidence, sat in front of me and, for the first time in a very long time, made no value judgements about me and what I ate.

She simply wanted me to understand why I did it, why I self-medicated with fresh bread, and why it was making me so unhappy.

She didn't need, or desire, any clarification, unlike me – I just wanted to be told just what to do to change my world. And it didn't start with the loaded sentence, 'Eat Less And Exercise More.'

I don't know how she did it, what suggestions she gave me to make me re-evaluate my perception of myself, but I just broke down in tears.

It was a mixture of embarrassment and wonder, to be honest. I sat there and, unable to stop, cried like the rain about it all.

Janet, bless her beautiful face and spiky hair, suggested that I wasn't entirely to blame for my, for want of a better word, predicament.

Gently, but assuredly, she nudged out of me stories about my childhood, how I ate adult portions with adult gusto with the adults at meal times, and got me to remember my particular – I'm avoiding the word peculiar here – bedtime stories.

It was like an 'Eureka!' moment for me, thinking that maybe, possibly, perhaps, dear God alive, I wasn't entirely to blame for my skewed relationship with food and, plodding along nicely now, myself.

But the guilt for thinking such things, for even giving headroom to the fact that those who loved me most could have aided and abetted my behaviour, almost killed me. And then came the tears.

I grew up in a loving house, where I was the two eyes in everyone's head. I could have what I wanted – within reason – so I was invariably given whatever I wanted to eat, and it was nothing for someone to come upstairs of an evening and ask me if I wanted a roll to go to sleep with. Yes, other people had teddies, I had a ham and tomato baguette.

My fab father would cut back on the time spent making one by freezing ham rolls and putting them in the microwave if I wanted a quick snack. In effect, I was rewarded for being good, for getting good marks, for being a clever bugger, for eating up all my dinner (and leaving my grancha's).

But to give these suggestions headroom? Well, it was like Janet was asking me to slap everyone who ever looked after me in the face and scream "abuser!"

I am an only child. Some people, with better resources, bigger eyes and obviously bigger brains than I have, apparently can tell that I am.

Whenever they say to me, "Ah, yes, I knew you don't have any brothers and sisters straight away", I have to stop myself from asking them if the word SELFISH is tattooed on my forehead, to go along with the PORKER written in invisible Indian ink on my knuckles.

What is it about me that says "She's Never Had To Share", I wonder? Janet knew I didn't have any siblings straight away, bright spark that she was.

She got me wondering if there is a little quirk I display which indicates that I grew up around adults, found other kids largely boring, and had to content myself with my own company for hours on end?

I can honestly say, however, that I don't think I missed out on sharing my family life with a sibling, another version of me, while I was growing up.

Sure, company would have been nice, chopsing about the folks, to someone who also benefited from their brand of tough love, on occasion may have been beneficial in a letting-off steam kind of way.

But I can't say that I longed for a sibling and that's

possibly because, as those sages say, you can't miss something you've never had.

As I've grown older, I've not grown whimsical. I'm just someone who's 34, childless and single, who simply doesn't have someone with similar DNA to share memories with.

What this means is, I don't have someone, other than my parents, to look back with.

And you know what? I couldn't care less.

I wanted for nothing as a child – emotionally speaking – and was lavished with attention. Then Janet pointed out to me that not wanting for anything food wise may – tiny word with big consequences that 'may' – have contributed to me eating my willpower in later life.

Emotionally speaking, it wasn't the kind of attention that blinded my parents to my many shortcomings; neither was I spoiled in a brazen, Violet Elizabeth kind of way. That's not my style, and pandering wasn't theirs.

But I will admit to missing, in those days when I felt utterly lonesome, and had grown out of standing on a bar stool in our pub singing 'Long-Haired Lover From Liverpool' to what were affectionately known as the Rhymney Boys, to get money for pop and crisps, someone cut from the same cloth – kid company.

I wanted, in those rare and needy moments, to put on shows with my brother (it was always a brother in my mind) and think, when I was getting in a row for setting fire to Uncle Ray's shed (he was a coal merchant and pal Liam and I were cold!) that I wasn't the only one in the firing line.

The closeness of siblings, that privileged position of being the constituent parts of a whole, was brought home to me this week after reading a story about actor Damian Lewis and his baby brother Gareth.

They shared ambitions and similar points of reference as they grew up, and they teamed up in a creative way to make a film together. They say it has brought them closer together.

Me? The only thing I made with my pretend now-and-again brother was a mess in the kitchen. And the only downside of making magic potions with Chanel No 5, a big bottle of Brut and shaving foam was that there wasn't anyone else around to share the blame.

Similarly, there wasn't anyone there to share the love. And, being a greedy only child, that has always suited me just fine. Besides, I could never think of anything worse than having to go halves on my slices of belly pork from Brynmawr market on a Saturday.

And maybe therein lies the root of my grown-up problems.

> # She looked as if she had been poured into her clothes and had forgotten to say "when"
>
> ### P.G. Wodehouse

I'VE NEVER MET ANY members of the Royal Family – and I'm not talking Caroline Aherne's lot either.

But I have been close. Well, when I say close what I actually mean is nowhere really near, at least not hand-shaking distance.

The first time I saw Prince Charles, he drove past me in a speeding car. So fast was he going up a hill in Ebbw Vale, that I was splashed with dirty steelworks' water and he was thrown around in the back, at not so much a jaunty angle, as a sack the driver one.

A Royal at a 45 degree angle isn't a pretty sight. But I admit it's rather a funny one.

Years later I was invited to a posh do where the guest of honour was the Queen.

This time I was so close – but I was still in the cheap seats – I could see her bra straps through her red satin dress.

Yep, bra straps.

Think here of a nan's thick straps holding her bits up under a not-so-nice all-in-one and you're somewhere close to its girth.

I also watched her out of the corner of my eye, wondering what she was like off-message.

Would she laugh? Would she find the turns on stage funny? Or would it be just another day at the office, albeit without a computer in front of her?

If you're interested, she squealed at Joe Pasquale, tapped her foot to 'Sit Down You're Rocking The Boat' but turned her head and looked around the venue when Katherine Jenkins came on in an electric dress. Yep, electric.

You should have seen the size of the plug and HM's short-lived surprise, no doubt wondering for a moment where they had put it in.

Anyway, I had to go to this do because it was work-related when, if I'm honest, I would rather have slid into a contented stupor on the white settee at home, my very favourite place to (literally) hang out (cheeky bugger Hiya Love says I only turn over on it every 20 minutes or so to avoid bed sores and to make sure my legs don't seize up).

Other people, though, members of the I'm Not Fat League for the Blind, Deaf and Stupid, don't get my reticence to go out, particularly to a big do such as HM's bash or the Baftas (yes, I've been and no, I didn't enjoy it).

It's a known fact that I don't like socialising much. Ask any of my patient friends.

I'm not fussed on schmoozing either – I can't do the 'Look At Me' thing, the showing off, the basic rules of socialising.

I'm also crap at being a certain somewhere filled with certain someones who know undeniable somethings about this and that – all of which you should know more about than you really do – and making light of the situation.

But I refuse to accept the Averageness of me, which, I think, becomes enlarged when surrounded by little black dresses topped off by faces which invariably look like someone's set them on fire and knocked them out with a cricket bat.

People don't notice faces, do they? They eye up firm bodies, though, they gaze at visible panty lines like salivating jealous puppies, they judge their own appeal by the size of someone's waistline.

I have an aversion to air-kissing and cheek-to-cheek caresses with strangers you wouldn't invite to a party even if the numbers were short.

That whole fashion statement of faux intimacy and familiarity tinged with the formality of stuffy manners is an odious concept to me.

But, saying that – here's the ironic bit – I pout and preen when I don't get invited to a fancy affair.

I don't know if I have a touch of the Dietrichs about me – the 'I vunt to be aloooone' syndrome – or that I'm just plain odd (no comments from the cheap seats, please).

But I often think that by not going to these VIP invite-only events an air of mystery will hang about me like an oblique cloud of intrigue, impenetrable but fascinating, just like ol' Marlene herself.

"Yeah, right – not when you come from the Rassau love!", the devil on my shoulder shouts.

In that curious place called Hannah World I tend to think that, when it comes to parties and launches and lunches, my 'aura' is made present by the lack of my physical presence. Know what I mean?

It's like that, by not being there, people will wonder why, so, in effect I will be noticed. Get it?

In reality, I imagine no one really gives a bugger if I'm out or not and, because I'm known in certain circles to be more reclusive than Howard Hughes, they wouldn't know me if I walked in wearing a rabbit suit or jumped out of a cake singing Agadoo.

So why do I find it so surprising when I don't get invited to attend the 'glamorous' side of my job?

This ball of confusion hit me again the other day when one of my colleagues asked me when Bafta Cymru was taking place.

Poised over his dairy with pen in hand, I gave him the date, assuming that he was just making a mental note to avoid Cardiff city centre on that particular day.

But no, he was writing it down because he wanted to find the place in his diary where he had made a note of the SEVEN invitations he had received to attend this year's ceremony.

I told him that I was still considering which invitation to accept.

What I didn't tell him was that I hadn't received even one to mull over at that point.

As disappointment started to stick in my throat I remembered that I went last year and it's not every day Jonathan Pryce asks you to pass the bread rolls.

I'm still waiting for the postman to bring me my plethora of invitations, so that at least I'll feel part of the establishment.

However, I'm far happier miles away from the action. A place where I can be – reluctantly perhaps – kind of invisible.

Thinking it over, who wants to be a nobody anyway? And that's what I would have been, a tiny and relatively badly dressed Welsh dot in the book of fame if I had gone to another do which I had a sniff of an invite to.

It's somewhat heart-warming to know that some parties are intimidating affairs, no matter who you are.

At a rather fancy advance screening of *Doctor Who* in Cardiff last year, filled to the brim with a galaxy of the BBC's biggest players, a certain award-winning actress was spotted arguing with her manager.

They weren't seen, you understand. A gaggle of journalists lapped it up by crowding around a toilet door as the designer-clad pair screamed at each other over the cubicles.

"You want to stop drinking and get out there now, you silly cow," said the manager.

A few monosyllabic threats were thrown back under the toilet door by the inebriated thespian, who promptly left the loo and landed smack-bang in the journo pack as she opened the door, and they unceremoniously fell onto her.

Then, regaining that smile and sense of sassy self that has made our secret gal a media darling, she grabbed the hand of her manager, sweetness and light restored once more, and said, "Come on girl, let's quit this place. There's an awful stench of PIG in here."

And with these words, she stormed back into the party battlefield very much, as someone there put it to me later, like Henry V at Agincourt. Only in high heels.

Granted, in Welsh terms, the *Doctor Who* do was a big deal, and people were largely on their best behaviour. But can you imagine the pressure you'd be under to perform if you were invited to the biggest bash of them all, the Oscars?

A few years back, S4C threatened to take me to LA if they were lucky enough to be nominated that year for an animated film. Sadly they weren't, but it was a lucky escape for me. Can you imagine ME at the Oscars?

I don't have a celebrity stylist and the only Oscar I know is that dirty fella who lived in a rubbish bin on Sesame Street.

Whereas others would have been shouting out to their celebrity friends as if reciting a diamond-encrusted rosary – "Angelina! Jim! Reese! Gwyneth! Julia!" – I don't think me going, "Little Dai! Big Dai! John Horse! Ted the Post! Hiya Love! Mam Jones!" has the same kind of pull.

I was also invited to the *Doctor Who* bash. Guess who didn't go?

Hey, when you can't imagine looking good enough to breathe the same air as Cher, you're on to a loser if fighting over the vol-au-vents with Billie Piper leaves you nervous.

Besides, what would I wear? It wouldn't have been a smile, I can tell you.

> **Americans can eat garbage, provided you sprinkle it liberally with ketchup, mustard, chilli sauce, Tabasco sauce, cayenne pepper, or any other condiment which destroys the original flavour of the dish**
>
> **Henry Miller**

I MISS AMERICA. I hope you didn't read that as I AM Miss America!

That simply wouldn't do.

No, I'm the newly crowned Miss Arse So Fat I Can Sit On A Rainbow And Make Skittles Come Out 2007 and my special interests are The Golden Girls, series one to three, the poems of e.e. cummings, the life, times and big thoughts of Jean-Paul Sartre and all-you-can-eat American-style buffets.

If we are what we eat, then I'm a steak and curly fries girl, piled high in a bid to satisfy the Desperate Dan side of Han; I'm melted cheese with burny bits skulking on the edges, I'm hot pretzels on a cold day, strawberry cheesecake at any time, all day breakfasts at midnight and always a stack of pancakes short of sated.

We Europeans may like to think of ourselves as cultured foodies, that it's quality not quantity that matters when it comes to a powerful and fulfilling dining experience.

But being what they call in the Valleys a gutsy bugger, I have to admit to being the polar opposite of this (burger) chain of thought.

In short, I was born to eat, drink and be merry in an American diner.

I am what you'd call a comfort eater, someone whose pleasure comes not from exquisite cuisine but in real soul food, only with less beans and gumbo.

I'll never forget my first visit to a diner in the US – they had Heinz red sauce on the table!

I don't mean a sachet of poor imitation red sauce, which is what I'd always found in restaurants in other countries, but the proper stuff (of course I didn't know then that it actually came from there in the first place).

The portions were huge, the taste incredible, the dessert menus straight from the fantasy scene of the cinema banquet in my mind.

My options included dough well done with cow to cover (that's buttered toast), a bowl of birdseed (cereal), a glass of drag one through Georgia (cola with chocolate syrup) to go with Noah's boy on bread (ham sandwich) from the soup jockey (waitress).

I just loved the way size really, really mattered for a change, served up in that way kids (or was it just me?) imagined table-buckling party food in heaven would look like.

Of course, I couldn't live in America – I'd be dead by now, crushed under the weight of a dream sequence of me and a load of Zeppelins in a fog while trying to make room for a certain Eve with a mouldy lid.

That's sausage and mash with a side of apple pie with a slice of cheese on top if you're interested.

Some would say, of course, that there's no need to go to America to eat like an American.

Yankee cuisine can be replicated in any British kitchen by mixing peanut butter with mashed up bananas, ladling it on toast and deep-frying it in lard until golden brown.

Mmm, just like Elvis used to make. And it didn't do him any harm.

Did it?

> **Some people change their ways when they see the light; others when they feel the heat**
>
> **Caroline Schoeder**

I'M BOILING. THE HEAT I can't do anything about, but I'm sure I could water down my frustration with myself if I were smaller.

I've no idea what that's like because even when I was smaller, I was still bigger than average, and always bigger than I was before I noticed I was getting bigger again! Keeping up? If only I'd settled for being a size 18 then a 20 then a 22 and a comfortable 24.

At each fleshy juncture, however, I did that old routine of feeling decidedly dissatisfied with myself and falling into the trap of trying to diet, trying to exercise, and landing flat on my bum each and every time – the only upside being that it's well-cushioned.

Of course, from there I became even more frustrated and ate my IQ in nonsense – and I'm a clever girl, me, except where it comes to counting calories, that is.

In the area of self-acceptance I'm also a veritable retard, a single cell above an emotional amoeba, someone who doesn't live for today but dreams of better tomorrows.

In the end, I'm really not much of a dreamer. I'm a realist trapped in the body of a faux-fantasist, someone who suffers at her own pudgy hands until I get to the point when even looking in the mirror is a chore because I know what I'll see there. But according to those who know me it's not what the rest of the world sees. In that case, I need laser surgery.

Of course, I can rumble on for ages thinking I'm OK, convincing myself that today – TODAY – is the day I will finally come to terms with being, well, me. That today – anyone got a calendar? – is the day I will get real about myself (sue me, I've been reading a Dr Phil book).

And then I sweat.

Then I get pissed off with myself. Then I recall I don't have any summer tops. Then I think that if I buy them, they won't come with sleeves. Then I think I can't possibly be seen without sleeves. Then I think about shoes, how much I hate shoes, wondering where I can get lessons in wearing flip-flops or those floppy mule things with sparkly bits on that sound as if women are dragging a suitcase when they walk.

Then I sweat some more.

Then I wear my slippers to work, convincing myself everyone will think they're mules. Then I get depressed about that.

Then I get home, take off my bra, step barefoot onto a cool wooden floor, pull on my comfies, and try to forget my displeasure at my crushing inability to feel comfortable with my place in the world – by turning to the fridge.

Then I think, oops, the cycle's started again.

The other day I was so hot, bothered and down about the slippers episode – yes, I really did wear them to work – that I mused on the whole thing by nibbling on a crisp sandwich WHILE waiting for my chicken to cook for a fat-free salad.

How's that for calorie-confused irony?

Salads are good, fabulous, tasty, wonderful – but not when a full sized one is used as the dessert in my crazy dinner party for one. So as I boil, bake and fry (I normally grill, girls – honest) I once again beat myself up about two things which vie for my attention.

First up is my inability to say to myself, bugger it, you're fine.

Second, is my round and round, stop and start approach to healthy living that never gets me anywhere apart from increasingly frustrated and self-critical.

Why can't I say to myself that I'm fabulous *now*, right this second, on this day and every day hereafter?

Maybe it has something to do with the heat – or a leak I have in my head that makes me feel totally unfabulous precisely because I've not got the tools I need to think any other way.

Being big means I can't strip off, bare all, and jump under a waterfall in a skimpy bikini like weathergirl Lisa Lloyd-Hughes did the other day.

I wasn't jealous of her beauty, but I get heartbroken when I can't display this sense of bodily freedom most slim girls seem to be born with.

I'm boiling. And today I'm boiling mad with myself for covering up, not only my arms, to this life of mine.

Is there chicken in chickpeas?

Helen Adams

I'VE DONE SOMETHING MOMENTOUS today – I've had just one (count it) piece of toast for breakfast.

Hey, I've HAD breakfast, which is a feat in itself.

People who eat 'normally' are under the false impression that all we foodies do is eat non-stop.

In fact, nothing could be further from the truth.

The other day I went to pal Andrea's hen do at a Greek restaurant. Now being as adventurous with food as I am with extreme sports, the idea of uncooked cheese and olives (eh? the point please?) just doesn't make me happy. I mean I come from a home where gravy is also an after-dinner treat.

But I went – and spent £20 on four chips and a pint of diet Coke.

I didn't eat a thing, save the four chips; I just sat there prodding and poking my food, smelling it (I always eat with my sense of smell and sight, before taste), trying to work out what the hell had been put in front of me.

But not liking stuff never worries me because I'm used to going places and not liking anything at all.

This bloke took me out for dinner once and I laughed to myself when I read the menu, without a single thing listed being suitable for this simple girl with simple tastes.

He ended up with plates filled with fancy grub, the names of which I couldn't pronounce.

The proprietor felt so sorry for me that he went up to

his living quarters, opened up his freezer and got his chef to cook me some of his children's faves.

So there we were, him with a colourful array of pigeon, jus and a medley of some discordant veg, while I'm nibbling on chicken nuggets and alphabet-shaped potatoes.

Anyway, my point is that being a limited foodie, but still a foodie in the non gastronomic sense, I can go for days without eating a thing.

Food fascinates me – equally, it bores me.

Unlike people who have a healthy relationship with it, being thwarted by it doesn't embarrass me.

So while I'm content to make four chips last all night in the Greek place, my pals are oohing and aahing all around me, worried that I'm not eating anything and getting worked up by it.

But to someone who had three courses of bread and butter in two different Michelin-starred restaurants, four chips felt like I was feeding an army.

I was also having one of my uninterested days, when food didn't matter. I left the restaurant unsatisfied but not hungry, and the next morsel I had was at least 24 hours later.

This week I'm off to the Significant (thin) Other's house, who is coming out in a worry rash wondering what to cook for me, what food to buy, what to treat me to.

The trick here, of course, is not to draw attention to my foodie shortcomings and then try not to make myself depressed when it becomes an issue for the host.

If you invite me round and I don't nibble, don't worry – at least you'll know I'm not going to fade away and radiate.

But I warn you now – I'll feel better without feta.

> **Nobody would be a celebrity if they weren't severely damaged. We're just looking for all the love we never got as children. Nobody should look up to us, we're basically circus freaks**
>
> **Roseanne Barr**

I WAS NEVER ONE of those kids with posters of pop stars on my wall. Not that I didn't like the Bay City Rollers or want to be Suzi Quatro, mind you.

While friends of mine hankered after looking like Kim Wilde, I was far too busy trying to sound like her – you know, like you've got the flu.

But if someone told me I could skip a few meals and get that Sandra Dee look – the black-clad vixen one Olivia Newton-John had going on at the end of Grease – I would have gladly given up my Desperate Dan-sized plates of steak and chips at Chez Jones for a while.

Now let me get this clear.

I'm not advocating that all bright young wannabes should skip meals to look like their idea of perfection.

But surely there's nothing wrong with a little bit of dreaming?

Take Atomic Kitten's Natasha Hamilton for instance.

The poor girl sparked one hell of a fury among parents and dieticians when she claimed the secret to her slim figure was not eating three meals a day. Big wow.

The former Rear of the Year was then asked how she got her figure back so quickly after the birth of her son

Joshua.

With fans clinging to her every word she responded candidly, "That's easy, I just don't eat. That's how I've done it. The way to a nice backside is not to eat."

Honest. What a great answer – no bullshit, no glossing, just plain facts.

Although a spokesman for Atomic Kitten later said the singer's remarks had been intended as a joke and she had corrected herself by saying her figure was down to a fast metabolism, her ill-judged comment caused outrage among watching parents.

Why, though? As far as I can tell she was just telling it like it is for her, not setting down the 11th Commandment, for all young girls to live by.

People wouldn't get in such a moral muddle if they lived balanced lives and didn't take every star's word as gospel.

I mean, they're not known for their brain power are they? And often they're all the better for it.

Our Tash wasn't playing up – or down – to the media machine when she said what she did.

And, thankfully, nor was she worrying about taking responsibility for the hordes of teens out there who take what members of pop bands say very seriously indeed.

It's not her job to preach to kids – that's the role of parents who have to make sense of what celebs do and say and put it into context.

I knew, for instance, that I'd never be Doyle from *The Professionals* (but it took an adult to tell me, kindly, that I had the wrong bits and was an only child).

I realised Purdy was Joanna Lumley playing a role as soon as someone took me aside and told me that putting a sieve on my head and cutting round it would not make me look like her.

As for Sandy, well, I decided to start eating my steak and chips again after a look at myself in the mirror, while pulling on skin-tight leggings proved to me that no amount of meal skipping would disguise my belly.

And I enjoyed every mouthful – while still holding on to the dream that one day I could be just like Kim and Purdy and Jimmy et al.

Like I said, we can all dream.

Fat-free beef dripping anyone?

No one can make you feel inferior without your permission

Eleanor Roosevelt

I HAD A CALL from someone the other day who said my newspaper column is a waste of time.

The person (and PLEASE don't call me again to say you read this remark and to give me another talking to about my limitations as you see them) said it wasn't doing anybody any good, it was giving the wrong message to women and that I was – am – basically a lazy, defeatist cow with nothing good to say.

Oh, but still 'quite nice looking' apparently. Ladies and gentleman, thank you and good night – he's got the measure of me and I'm bowing out.

Nah, not really, but I couldn't help but think he had a point.

However, I don't think he quite grasped that the column is attempting to be entertaining as well as an open letter to myself.

It's a slight – only slight – exaggeration of what is, otherwise, a rather dull life spent, largely, trying to come to terms with myself. But it IS about me, about what I think, what I do, how I see myself and so on. It's not easy reading sometimes – hey, it's not easy writing at ANY time – but it is honest.

That said, I do ask myself how many times I can openly berate myself in this way; how many times I can chart what I ate or didn't eat; and the battle I have with exercise and self image. But – here's a thing for my detractors to think about – people are always contacting me to tell me they like it.

Don't ask me why, and don't ask me how – that's like asking me to draw one of those silly charts and put down on one side what I think is just fabulous about me. I might get as far as line two, but that's about it on the plus side.

What I can do, because my glass is always half full, with a chip on the lip and a crack up the side, is what people tend to shy away from, and that's expressing what it's like to be in my skin and inside my head.

And that often isn't pretty.

This is me, warts'n'fat'n'all. It's me – Hannah the defeatist, the optimist, the dieter, the girl who says bugger that for a laugh, the mass of contradictions that makes me, well, me. If that confirms me as self-indulgent, so be it – I didn't ask for this gig, but now I'm here I'm not going to fold because someone believes I'm as much use as a chocolate ashtray, or a condom machine in the Vatican toilets.

Frankly, I don't need anyone to tell me that, or to read it in six foot flashcards. As they say in Cardiff, "I knows what I knows, love."

Anyway, the person who called me is a fitness trainer who has, I'm sure, my best intentions at heart.

What I can't stand, however, is people like him talking to me like I'm just a positive thought away from mending myself. I know that to lose weight I have to obliterate my portions, eat less, exercise more, and start to think straight.

I just don't know how to maintain that level of interest in myself.

Do you?

I'm not talking the kind of interest that tells you your fringe needs a tidy-up, or you must go out shopping for a new pair of shoes. I mean real life-altering stuff: where you start to think clearly and stop defining yourself by a series of numbers on scales, and you don't take umbrage at someone who thinks writing about your endless jaunt on this dead-end journey is a waste of time.

I'm with him on that to be honest – but even my silence won't stop my struggle to be a better version of what's singularly known as Me.

Because as Mam Jones often reminds me, "It's rude not to share."

Read all about it, or turn away. It's really quite simple – a lot easier than calorie counting, I can tell you.

> **No fashion has ever been created expressly for the lean purse or for the fat woman: the dressmaker's ideal is the thin millionairess**
>
> **Katherine Fullerton Gerould**

JUST BECAUSE SOMETHING IS in fashion, it doesn't mean it's advisable to wear it. Here's the low-down on what we bigger girls should be buying and shying away from…

1. Dogtooth patterns

AVOID. The only dog I want to see about my person is my Jack Russell, Bertie, on a lead. This trend is a load of rubbish and is bound to date. DO NOT make the mistake of thinking that just because thinnies think this is 'in', you have to follow suit.

2. Long knitted jumpers

Hmmm… debatable. Do you really want to add extra inches in chunky knitwear? Go for it if you're quite tall, but avoid it if you're more short, fat and dumpy than long-legged and lovely. I'd go for a swishy wrap instead to keep me warm.

3. Navy blue colours

Ship ahoy! No problem with dark colours at all. Don't

make the mistake of wearing light-coloured trousers and tops together. This big girl I know had on a white fluffy jumper and cream cords the other day – honest to God, she looked so ridiculous that when kids saw her they came running out of their houses with carrots because they thought it'd started snowing.

4. Ochre and red

Oh autumn… a time for reflection, a time for dancing in the rain, not a time for muted colours. Be brave with colour, but don't plaster yourself in it. And ONLY do it up top – always keep your trousers or skirts dark, preferably black and wide-legged if you're going down the trousers route.

5. Mustard

Can't stand it in sandwiches and I certainly don't like it in clothes. After all, who wants to look like a giant sun gone wrong? If you want to wear colour, opt for pastel shades instead. Don't run the risk of thinking you've got it going on in gone off yellow. BIG mistake.

6. Leggings

If they're good enough for Madonna, they're good enough for us. Right? WRONG! They're basically tights with the feet cut off. The 80s are long gone, and good riddance I say. If you're feeling nostalgic, get some shoulder pads. At least your waist will look smaller.

7. Buttons

In the same way that life is too short to change gears in a car, I'd say it's also too short to spend your time doing up buttons. Slimmies might think they look fab in a Twiggy kind of way and believe that it's OK to put big buttons on neck lines, but remember that less is more. If you're going to wear them, make sure they're in the colour of your clothes and not like oversized Smarties in rainbow colours.

Ooh, Smarties – lush! Sorry, where was I?

> **It's OK to be a fat man. It's prestige and power and all of that. But fat women are seen as just lazy and stupid and having no self-control**
>
> **Camryn Manheim**

I'M BACK FROM A week in Ireland. Not that I like holidays much, you understand – they're too much like hard work.

Perhaps that's a slight exaggeration, but I honestly don't find living out of a suitcase very enjoyable.

Nor do I like the tense, nervous headache I get when boarding a plane and wondering if the seat belt will go around me (check) or if I have to pretend my baby is sitting with its father 15 rows back because we had a row – "he called me fat because he said I was so big I'd have to make two flights to get where we're going" (sob) – so I can get an extension?

Trust me, I had the conversation in my mind with the invisible father of my non-existent child just in case I had to make up an excuse for my belly on the spot.

Shame they didn't give out badges for quick thinking in the Brownies.

Anyway, as a Sagittarian, I'm supposedly a free-spirited gal who likes to travel. I should have been born under a different star sign because, to be truthful, I'm neither.

But when I was offered 'a trip of a lifetime' to Canada last year to review a show that was coming to Wales, I thought I'd better show willing, if only to prove I hadn't been born under a wandering star.

The trip was fraught with difficulties from the beginning, but I reassured myself that Canada being a nation of pancake lovers would make up for the pain. Only learning where I would be staying on the morning of my flight, I sat waiting patiently in the departure lounge of Cardiff International Airport.

And then it all started to go horribly wrong; the sound of the bing-bong all travellers hate to hear, "We're sorry but the flight to Amsterdam is delayed."

No problem, I thought at first. Huge problem, I thought two hours later.

Because when I eventually arrived in Amsterdam to catch my connecting flight to Montreal, I was informed by a flight attendant with a PhD in perfect make-up that my plane was leaving as we spoke. Oh, and my luggage was also 'enjoying Britain' i.e. still on Welsh soil.

Said Thing of Beauty then told me to "hurry my little legs up" as a flight was leaving for – shock horror – Detroit in 15 minutes' time.

So off I ran – well, ambled if I'm honest – sans luggage but with a migraine now, to Gate 24.

I checked in and was frisked, prodded and poked. I eventually got to the right departure gate only to be told in the international language of sign that I was FIVE HOURS EARLY for the flight to Detroit and that I wouldn't be allowed back out to buy a can of Coke or fridge magnet in the shape of a windmill. And there wasn't a vending machine in sight.

Anyway, to cut a long story short, I got to Canada in the early hours of Saturday, 12 hours later than I should have got there, via America.

At 2a.m. Canadian time I went to find someone who could tell me about my lost luggage.

I was told it would be delivered to me – but that the

first flight to Montreal didn't land until 5p.m. that day. So I made my way to the hotel, one of the top 500 places to stay in the world, apparently, staring depressedly at TWO walk-in wardrobes with nothing to hang up in them.

Someone in the hotel said I could buy suitable 'lingerie' at a nearby chemists. But I doubted they'd do size 24 knickers off the rack.

This thought naturally made me even more fractious – I mean, if I was 'normal'-sized, lost undies wouldn't be a problem and I could easily find some cheap clothes to tide me over. Right?

Instead I was left fuming and feeling like I was buzzing as I mused on my inability just to make do. Big girls can't simply 'make do' unless Julie Andrews is on hand with some curtains and a sewing kit.

A day later, I'm back in the airport heading for home, having had my luggage returned to me a few hours before flying back.

With a few more minutes to kill I decided to check my email.

I follow the ENGLISH instructions and slot in my credit card, my ONLY source of money at that moment, and, you guessed it, it got stuck.

I phoned the help number with the few cents I had left – how I ached to spend them on more pancakes – and the second death-knell sounded with "our office opening hours are nine to five, Monday to Friday." This was 4p.m. Sunday.

After phoning my mother to tell her to cancel the card, I eventually found someone on the information desk who, before handing me the supposed answer to my prayers, gave me a tissue to wipe my teary eyes.

Now I must have an honest face as she gave me – I

kid you not – a letter opener the size of a machete.

There's only one snag, she said – if airport security saw me with said weapon, I'd be arrested for carrying it! She wrapped it up in a duster and told me to shove it up my coat sleeve.

So there I was, walking around the airport like a starving Spiderman ready to weave his web, but to no avail – the card wouldn't budge. Anyway, a construction worker eventually got it out with a pair of pliers, I called my mother to tell her not to cancel the card after all – she already had.

Before things could get any worse, I got on the plane – only for the bloke next to me to spill his orange juice over my passport, book and clothes. I went to the toilet and turned said clothes inside out and wore them like that all the way home, tags on show, and all.

I got to Cardiff, starving from the lack of plain food, with only the thought of stopping at Burger King on the drive home keeping me going.

And then came that blasted tannoy announcement again, "Ladies and gentlemen, sorry for the delay in getting you off this plane today. It appears that we can't find a pair of steps to fit the aeroplane."

Whispers from the trolley dollies – but sadly no free nuts – that the emergency slides might have to be deployed to get us out were thankfully unfounded.

Can you imagine what was going through my mind about deployment, suction, getting stuck and deflation, in more ways than one?

Rumours that I'm the love child of Alan Whicker and Judith Chalmers are, therefore, untrue.

Things weren't quite so bad on my latest trip, but the airport staff did manage to lose my luggage again. So I had to traipse around in manky jeans for two days out of four, feeling like the back end of a dirty Welsh bus.

The PR people had booked us into two of southern Ireland's fanciest hotels. With fancy rooms, as we all know, comes fancy grub; with fancy grub, comes me going "what the fuck am I going to do with orange and thyme confit duck leg, garlic pommes purées and hoi-sin sauce?"

I tell you another thing I don't quite get, and that's silver service. Can you believe there are some people out there who want to be served their selection of charcuterie, tossed salad and mixed pickles (dear God alive...) with backward-held spoons and forks? It's just another way for food to become ritualised and stuffy in my book, as something conceited rather than filling.

Anyway, once my luggage was returned and I could successfully dress for dinner (again, shouldn't that be a choice you make rather than a condition of getting a seat?) I ended up spending more time reading the menu than actually eating the food.

When we finally found a place which had (in rough translation) steak and chips, I thought there is a God after all.

But, to be honest, I couldn't wait to get home to a nice Sunday dinner (on a Wednesday) and know I wouldn't be expected to eat smoked salmon for breakfast and put a ball gown on just for pleasure.

On this mini-break I didn't really get to try many firsts.

On the plus side, I didn't have to worry about pleading for seconds either.

Or sewing six pairs of Medium-sized knickers together to 'make do'.

> **The second day of a diet is always easier than the first. By the second day, you're off it**
>
> **Jackie Gleason**

I'M HAVING A PARTICULARLY bad few days. From my shapelessly cut hair and its fading fake red colour, the same old make-up that doesn't seem to stay on my face longer than a heartbeat, to the clothes that scream dull; things externally aren't looking that good.

I'd have my hair cut – but, honestly, I can't bear to think about being sat in that bloody chair, in front of that bloody mirror, being asked by a bloody perfect specimen of salon chic in high heels if I'm going out tonight. Umm, no. Just to save time later.

I'd dye it, get rid of my roots (which look really odd as they're quite fair) but I can't muster the energy.

I've even got a 40% discount card for Evans, so buying some new clothes shouldn't be a big financial problem. I just can't seem to find the energy to be interested in myself. Of course, I've got all the oomph in me to feel despondent, discouraged and disappointed – that's never, ever, a problem.

But looking on the bright side of Me or even the semi-lit one is an uphill struggle. And as I said before, I'm built for comfort and not speed so I don't care much for inclines. Yawn.

Anyway, as if I wasn't feeling bad enough, someone at work – the same person who looked at a not-so-attractive slimmie then at me and said, "I bet you're really pissed off that you've got a great face and she's got a great body... isn't it a shame you can't have her figure, as she's an ugly cow," – turned to me last week and said, "Yes, I think you're right what you're saying. I am a fattist."

Now ordinarily I would have either laughed or wanted to punch him in the face. At that moment, though, because my defences were down and I was feeling like the poster child for misery, I looked at him and said, "Oh. OK. Want a cup of tea?" Biggies like me, girls who fluctuate from OK to Don't Even Ask Me What I Weigh, sometimes feel worthless, see. And that day was one of those occasions.

Our exterior body dysphoria dirties our self image until we're just shadows (as if!) of our former selves, (non) shrinking violets who can't quite put their fat fingers on what they need to do to stop the negative thinking and launch into life-changing action.

Oh, that's right – stop eating so much and move more. Quick! I've found the answer girls!

Yeah, right. Today, as my disappointment at my inability to be anything other than a lazy fat ugly cow rages (no letters, please), I'm managing to worship at the altar of a 21-year-old woman who's shed almost half her body weight after being too embarrassed to ask for size 28 clothes, wondering how the hell she managed to maintain enough interest in the process to do it.

Melissa Harrison, from Mansfield, Nottinghamshire, dropped from 19st 4½lb to 10st 3lb in 18 months and has been crowned Slimming World's Female Young Slimmer of the Year.

She said that before she lost weight she felt disgusted and disappointed with herself (check) but her confidence was too low to do anything about it (double check, underline, put in italics and highlight in yellow).

While her friends went out and enjoyed themselves (notice a theme here, said fingering an imaginary moustache?) Mel stayed at home hiding behind a mask of make-up and anger. She said she hated meeting new people because she thought they would be judging her (ain't that the truth).

But when her size 26 clothes began to feel too tight, and she realised the next pair of trousers she bought would have to be size 28, she decided it was time to act. She said, "I was disgusted with how big I had let myself get. I wasn't happy with my life and who I was so I thought it was time to do something about it.

"I didn't want to go out at night with my friends. Even when I was shopping, I would have to have someone with me in the hope that people would look at the other person rather than me.

"But even then, my friends would be buying nice little outfits and all I could try on was the jewellery."

She decided to join her local Slimming World group and 18 months later has succeeded in her dream of losing half her bodyweight.

Mel, who celebrated her win with a night out at celebrity haunt The Met Bar in central London, followed by a meal (hooray!) at Michelin-starred restaurant Nobu, said her diet of take-aways, chocolate, crisps, pies and butter (NOT guilty on this one) had caused her weight to spiral.

She shed 9st 1½lb and shrunk to a size 10 (eh?) after swapping her love of fast-food for healthier options. Mel said she followed an eating plan that allowed her to enjoy an unlimited amount of foods low in energy density such as pasta, rice, potatoes and lean meat.

It even permitted her to indulge in her favourite meal – a roast dinner. On one trip to the cinema, as her friends tucked into a bucket of sugary popcorn, she produced a roast chicken to snack on.

With her dramatic weight-loss, Mel said she has found a new confidence and happiness and is an inspiration to her friends.

"I can now do anything I ever wanted to do. I am living my life and very much enjoying myself," she said. "I go out and feel a lot more confident meeting new people. Before, I didn't want to talk to people I didn't know because I thought they would judge me, but I am very happy with who I am now. I am up for anything – any challenge I am happy to take on."

I just hope she didn't spend the £2,000 prize money on pizzas. Because today, looking and feeling like this, I fear that's exactly what I would do.

> **I've been on a Slim-Fast diet. For breakfast you have a shake. For lunch you have a shake. For dinner you kill anyone with food on their plate**
>
> **Rosie O'Donnell**

DADDY OR CHIPS? FAT-BUSTERS or Porkers-R-Us?

These are big conundrums for a big girl. Last week, while my trousers felt like I'd borrowed them from a three-year-old, I had a brainwave.

Nope, not to accept myself the way I am, wobbly bits'n'all, but to join a slimming club.

I thought the ritual humiliation every week of standing on the scales while women behind you contort to see the extent of the damage might put me on the right track.

But, being tight-fisted and a natural born defeatist, I thought I'd see if I could blag myself a membership. That way, I reasoned, I could write about my mishaps and mayhems and plug the diet, done by a real person with a hole in their head.

Fat Busters was approached via its press office and I set out the facts for them – you give me a membership and I, all size 24 of me, would write about my experiences of it in my 'Diary of a Diet' every week.

Two weeks later and I was still dipping white bread in the pasta sauce while waiting for my main meal to cook. In other words, they didn't get back to me.

So I took my life in my hands and called my local Fat Busters consultant and she told me about the timings of a class near to me (not very enthusiastically, I might add).

122

There I was, all ready to start last week, when I got an email through from Porkers-R-Us offering me six months of free access to their slimming site.

So, I face a big fat, thigh-chafing dilemma.

On the one hand I would have to do something ON MY OWN (nightmare) and follow the online stuff to the letter. Oh, but it would be free (pass me a Yorkshire pudding and a vat of my mother's gravy to celebrate). Or I could PAY to go to a class.

Significant (thin) Other advised me to go to the class, thinking that I'd be more likely to 'stick at it' if I was duty bound to go (how long has he known me now?).

Mam Jones, knowing that my dedication rate is in minus points when it comes to dieting and fitness, told me to do what I wanted (but reminded me of my overdraft limit).

Friend Justin (a fellow battler who's yo-yoed more times than a, er, yo-yo) told me to try the freebie one for six months and, if that didn't work, to go to the class.

So that's what I'm doing. I started the online thing a few days ago, trying to work out what my daily allowance of food meant in relation to sandwiches or pasties.

To be honest, I was pleasantly surprised because I ate well for the first few days and – if I was doing it right – I was about five points under each day. What's that about, then? By that reasoning I SHOULD be losing weight by just doing what I do normally. Right?

Wrong. My trouble is that, like Little Britain's slimming expert Marjorie Dawes, I live on dust.

Then I don't. Then I do. Then I don't again. I fluctuate from the sensible to the ridiculous with such crazy regularity that all my good intentions can melt in the damaged fridge-freezer of my mind in an instant – and just like my penchant for frozen cheesecake when I'm 'in a mood', I don't wait for my feelings to defrost.

The last time I went to a slimming class, the Marjorie Dawes of my youth (and there've been a few, I can tell you), had the scale set up to say "One at a time please" if you put on weight. The philosophy there, of course, was to embarrass and shock us all into doing better.

That failed with me and I was straight up to the Pizza Pan, in Ebbw Vale, for a cheese, onion, ham and mushroom delight which I nibbled while musing on being a pig. So maybe Porkers-R-Us, online and at home and also on the PC at work, will be better suited to me.

I just hope I don't get any viruses. Or the munchies.

> **The hatred of fat people, I think, is more modern. It's manufactured. It's a manifestation of the shabbier and cheaper side of culture, which is to say, advertising and skinny models on the beach hawking cigarettes and beer**
>
> **Daniel Pinkwater**

MY BEST FRIEND NICOLA has just come back from a trip to Belfast where she's realised one of her life's ambitions. She's gone back to Ebbw Vale fulfilled after apparently doing something with a Giant and his Causeway (I didn't ask, she's an adult after all), something, no doubt, that you need stamina and a waterproof jacket for.

She's just got walking on a glacier, going to see the mid-Atlantic ridge being born in Iceland, visiting Yellowstone National Park and the icebergs in Patagonia to go. Whereas all I want is to die knowing that once – just the once you understand – I've walked past Greggs and NOT gone in for a cold (it's got to be cold) cheese and onion pasty and a packet of five yum-yums.

There's also that little matter of self-acceptance to hanker after, but I'm talking about things I want to achieve in THIS life, not the next 20 reincarnations.

I also want to get through the day without someone asking me what I think about skinny people. Here's an answer for you – I think they're lucky cows.

I find my opinion on skinny models is being sought more than ever after *The Clothes Show Live* announced plans to ban 'stick-thin' models from the catwalk at its next show in December.

There's also that little matter of Spain's top fashion show turning away a number of models on the grounds they are too skinny – an unprecedented swipe at body images blamed for encouraging eating disorders among young people.

When I was young I didn't want the body of a model – I just wanted to feel, well, normal; to look normal. I didn't hanker after size 6 hips or being a boobless wonder. I simply wanted to go into a shop and buy the same things that my more 'normal'-sized friends had access to.

Today, I'm still the same. Frankly, I don't give a bugger if designers use size zero models – however, I don't quite get it.

Nor do I get it when catalogues, which sell clothes up to a size 34, picture nice-looking size 10 women in the stuff. Isn't that like advertising a holiday in Cannes with a picture of a seven-berth caravan in Porthcawl?

Both are nice, but they are different. Agreed?

So where will it all end? Should there be positive discrimination against women under a size 18 who want to work in Evans? Don't be silly – I mean, they always need thinnies to run up the stairs, rummage in the stock room for a smock top, and get down again quickly without the aid of an asthma pump.

The point I'm making is really quite simple – the fashion industry just needs to reflect that women come in all shapes and sizes (normally in double figures).

Don't stone me, but I honestly think that smaller women look better in fancy clothes. There, said it.

However, if they don't know what suits them and they fall foul of the laws of fashion and become victims, they'd better wish they had a bit of fat to hide behind. At my size I can't get away with cropped tops, tight clothes, high-waisted trousers, dainty underwear or tailored suits.

As a size 24 with opinions and eyes in my not so little head, I can see that I could get away with more and know more about what's out there if I had access to more role models who dress well and who, basically, don't give a shit about their limitations.

I don't get out of bed for less than $10,000 a day

Linda Evangelista

I'LL LET YOU INTO a little secret that only a handful of people know – I was once asked to be a model. No, not for fridge-freezers but for actual, proper, grown-up stuff like magazines, catalogues and – gulp – the catwalk.

OK, you can stop laughing now. I was at university and at a size 18-20 with a fabulous asymmetrical red bob, I didn't look that bad.

Of course, all I could see were the floppy bits, the bits I couldn't cover and that caused me such agony. Luckily, I had a friend who thought I wasn't bad-looking (then) and had an iota of fashion sense (I'm glad she can't see me now).

So, on the sly, she sent some pictures of me to a London model agency that specialised in (hold your sides just in case they split from laughing) 'plus-sized' girls.

Imagine my shock, horror and secret elation when they wrote back to me saying they 'loved' my picture and wanted to sign me up. Me! A model! Yep, hilarious.

But I am talking niche market here remember, not Models One – more like the Yes, That's Her Size Not Her Phone Number agency.

To be honest, the main reason I didn't accept is that I thought people would laugh at me, say things like, "Look at her! She thinks she's nice-looking. I've seen better looking sides of beef. And smaller arses on a cow. A model? Model disaster you mean."

128

I was also uncomfortable with the notion that people would think I loved myself when, as we all know, I'm at odds with most of the constituent (flabby) parts that make me who I am.

Anyway, to cut a long story short I declined, but inclined my ability to consume vast amounts of carbs.

And now I've just written about this long-held little titbit in the column, that same old insecurity – worrying about how other people think I perceive myself – still jabs at me.

But what if I had accepted and not let myself get so tangled up in this skewed vision I have of myself?

Maybe, just maybe, I would be in the front row at London Fashion Week cheering on the next round of 'fleshy' models, real girls with real curves. And don't think I'm talking a size 14 either.

I may not have a GCSE in logic, but even this thickie can see the worth in the MUCH BIGGER picture.

My organs are too powerful... I manufacture blood and fat too rapidly

Robert Baldwin

FORGET CONDOMS, BEING FAT is an effective contraceptive. Having a few extra pounds – stones in my case – can keep you safe from straying hands and wrap you up in the kind of safety where you don't run the risk of someone telling you that they'd like you better if you were just a bit smaller.

The steely-eyed feminist in me would like to think that if someone said this to me, I'd be able to come back with a witty retort such as, "You of all people should understand that I am quite happy and satisfied to be in this body. And it's a known fact that given the chance, you would be too."

Or, "Wow, you're kidding! You're actually telling me I can actually change my body? I'm so shocked!"

I can just hear me saying something like this, and then watching myself crumble in the corner, crying out of sheer frustration.

Now that I have what's known in the trade as a 'significant other', I've started to do that thing where I wonder what he really thinks of me.

Not that I have any doubt that he thinks I'm fun, great company, fabulous, witty, clever and wide-eyed. He tells me so in no uncertain terms – and I hear these words and largely believe them, no problem at all.

But when it comes to the question of my attractiveness, no amount of assurance will do it.

I've known myself to say, "Are you sure, I mean absolutely positive, that you're not embarrassed to be going out with someone like me?"

And by 'someone like me' I mean someone who is the 'F' word (and I'm not talking Fabulous here either).

Yet no amount of praise, encouragement or gasps of "you look powerful and striking today, Miss Jones" has the clout to translate it into words I understand. It's all mumbo jumbo to me.

I had an American boyfriend once who said he thought I was beautiful and sexy blah blah – but for all his brains and Buddhist Californian sensibilities, he added that it was a 'challenge' getting used to my body.

"You're kidding," came my retort. "I'm big? Who knew! Thanks SO much for letting me know. Seems I've learned a lot today."

Needless to say, our love affair didn't last because I ended it. See, even big girls don't have to settle.

I met him on the internet, the first of many 'dates' I made online.

They've all been a bit crackers (apart from the present Mr Han who I met in cyberspace and who now fills my personal space with ease), but at least I've got some stories to tell. In no particular order: I've met a pop star, a BAFTA Award-winning film director, a former Mr Europe, David Brent's love child who worked in a paper clip factory in Slough, two high-powered lawyers, a fishmonger and an environmental scientist.

Speaking as someone who is a born sceptic, I didn't look at internet 'dating' – ugh – as a method of finding my one true love.

But as good old Mam Jones once said to me, "You're not going to find someone on the way to filling up your dishwasher, love."

Not that she liked the idea of me opening myself up to strangers on the web, but I batted back her concerned, "You don't know if they're who they say they are," with a tentative, "And I would if I met them in a more conventional way?"

The internet has proved to be very good at two things – selling shit and dating – which are, in fact, much the same thing.

Online, you are your own matchmaker. The only trouble is, what we want and what our looks and status can afford are two different matters.

And people are fattist. On every 'dating' site I've been on, they all asked what your body type is. And if you ticked 'bigger than average' or 'got a few pounds to lose', blokes simply would, in the words of Dionne Warwick, walk on by.

I thought, in all my naivety, I'd have no problems with cyber dating which is, really, casting your net on the Net and getting to know someone a bit better without having to leave the comfort of your computer or wash your hair.

You can write each other little messages and pretty soon you'll find out all sorts of interesting things about your 'date' – such as, they can't punctuate. Oh, and however ugly and forward thinking they are, what they're really after is someone not on the big side of small.

Another downside is that nobody is really compelled to tell the truth, and that's where athletes are really men with two left feet, and high-powered city types really drive an Asda truck for a living. And a 'few extra pounds' translates as 'shaves legs with lawn mower'.

Nothing wrong with either, but fantasy isn't my reality.

The new Mr Han makes me feel, on the surface at

least, that I have (said in a Beyoncé style) got it going on. It's a pity her songs of self-affirmation only last four minutes, however.

So I'm hoping he'll help me hear strutting music wherever I go, to the point where I'll remember to change the stuck record to the theme tune of my fabulously 'F' life forever.

Just doing it for today is a good start, though.

You don't have to be age 20 and Size Zero to be sexually viable or viable as a woman

Belinda Carlisle

THERE'S UPROAR AT THE moment about a new telly show which will challenge women to crash diet. No great shakes, I hear you cry – until I tell you the producers want women to diet until they've got down to a size zero.

That's ZERO. As in nothing. As in inconsequential. As in bloody bonkers.

The Channel 4 documentary is a 'super-skinny' version of *Super Size Me*, in which a film-maker spent 30 days eating junk food. In the 2004 film, Morgan Spurlock ate nothing but McDonald's meals for an entire month and his resulting physical and emotional decline was charted.

Those picked to go on this show, which will be called something like *Super-Skinny Me: The Race to Size Zero* – and they're all girls of course – will employ 'extreme weight-loss methods' to slim down. So far so good and I'm thinking, hey, where do I sign up to slim down?

But the downside of downsizing is that these guinea pigs will attempt to emulate Hollywood stars, such as the shockingly thin Nicole Richie, in the hour-long programme.

A US size zero – equivalent to our British size four – has become the holy grail for image-conscious celebrities. But not for me.

As I see it, most women want to lose weight. But if you're happy and you know it, and you really want to show it, at a super-size whatever, that's fine by me – I'd clap my hands along with you!

Nor would I mind a dieting show which had experts on hand to show me how to get the weight off really, really quickly – I mean, who has time for patience, right?

The point I'm making is that some people are happy with their bodies whatever their size, so they shouldn't be made to feel uncomfortable about it.

I would go on a diet show without hesitation. But at least I'd know when to stop. I mean, who in their right mind would *want* to be a size zero? It's bloody bonkers.

Who would like to go into a shop and ask, "Excuse me love, but do you do this in a size dot?"

I've never wanted to be anything other than a good old-fashioned size 16 – but that was my ambition when I was a 20. These days, at a size 24, I'm ever more realistic and a size 20 seems like my version of the holy clothes (g)rail.

I just don't get it when a girl who, at a size 14 wants to be a size 8. Or smaller. Why would anyone with their marbles intact want to forsake even a glimmer of curvaceousness for ramrod lines? Beats me, and I'm as messed up as the next person about my body image.

Anyway, back to the shock doc. A Channel 4 spokesman (of course it's a bloke) says the show has a "real sense of purpose" and that it "provides the perfect opportunity to debunk the current clamour for all things super-skinny."

Because, you see, it's apparently all for a good cause. Producers are being altruistic because what they're really trying to do is, no, not get women like me tuning in by the million to find out the quickest route to 'average', but to let the whole wide world know about the health dangers lurking behind radical weight loss.

Yeah right, and I'm Kate Moss's left thigh.

The Eating Disorders Association said it has "very serious concerns" about the health of the women taking part in the show. They've pointed out that extreme weight loss can lead to major medical problems and can affect fertility – tell that to someone who wants to buy skinny jeans and a cropped top. The association's spokesman, Steve Bloomfield, said that those picked to go on the show also run the risk of becoming addicted to the weight loss programme and developing eating disorders as a result.

"We certainly have very serious concerns about the health of the participants," he said.

"We know from research that even with those who voluntarily reduce their weight below a safe BMI (body mass index), there is the possibility they may actually develop anorexia because eventually the fasting becomes compulsive and the dieting becomes obsessive.

"It could be very difficult to eat normally again after the experiment is over.

"There are some potentially quite serious risks to the participants.

"Extreme weight loss can cause a woman's periods to stop and as little as three months without periods can lead to osteoporosis.

"If you burn off all your body fat then you start burning muscle – the heart is one of the biggest muscles in the body and you start running the risk of heart disease, which is a real issue for anorexics.

"We are not going to condemn a programme that we haven't seen but we would certainly like to see a very high level of close medical supervision for the participants."

Channel 4 defended the programme.

Their spokesman came back with, "This documentary will highlight the dangers of aiming for a 'super-skinny' look, and expose the serious health risks of extreme weight-loss methods, all of which are already in the public domain.

"At every stage of filming there will be continuous, full medical support and expert guidance at hand."

What do I think? Well, I'd go on. I'd endure the emotional ups and downs, the fasting, prodding, poking and cajoling and everything modern science could throw at me – but only until I hit that cherished size 16-18.

Then I'd walk. Odd I may be, but I do know when enough's enough (unless it comes in an all-you-can-eat Chinese buffet) without hitting rock bottom on my clothes tags.

Size Zero? You know where you can stuff it.

> **The devil has put a penalty on all things we enjoy in life. Either we suffer in health or we suffer in soul or we get fat**
>
> **Albert Einstein**

I'VE JUST BEEN GIVEN a new piece of advice – stop eating when you're full.

Good, isn't it? At last there's something I can follow, a tip from the top, a definitive perfect sense guide to building a better me. Not. Telling people not to eat when full is like telling an alcoholic to put down that cider, drink only in the evenings, and walk past their local Bargain Booze without going in. IT JUST DOESN'T COMPUTE. And don't just take my word for it, either.

Obese people are hooked on food in the same way drug addicts crave narcotics, new research suggests.

Brain circuits responsible for over-eating are the same as those involved in drug addiction, say scientists.

Researchers conducted brain scans of seven obese (how I hate that word) individuals fitted with 'gastric stimulators' – experimental implants designed to curb the appetite. Devices stimulate the stomach to send 'fullness' messages to the brain. Volunteers had scans to measure brain activity both with the stimulator on and off – but weren't told when they were switched on. Ooooh, sneaky.

Pinpointing the parts of the brain affected by the signals identified the 'gluttony' circuits, the team reported.

All that work for something I could have told Dr

Gene-Jack Wang – who led the research at the US Department of Energy's Brookhaven National Laboratory in New York – over a packet of crisps.

Dr Wang said, "We found that implantable gastric stimulators induced significant changes in metabolism in brain regions associated with controlling emotions, effectively shutting down these obese subjects' desire to eat." Keeping up? Hungry yet?

The effect was especially pronounced in the hippocampus brain region, where activity was 18% higher during gastric stimulation. The hippocampus is linked to emotion, learning and memory, and the processing of sensory and motor impulses. It also plays a role in the retention of memories related to drug experiences in addicts.

Satiety messages also activated brain circuits in the orbito-frontal cortex and striatum. These regions have been linked to craving in drug-addicted patients.

Participants were also questioned on three aspects of eating behaviour: cognitive restraint, uncontrolled eating and emotional eating.

When the gastric stimulator was switched on, 'emotional eating' – that's what I do – scores were 21% lower than when it was turned off.

"This provides further evidence of the connection between the hippocampus, the emotions, and the desire to eat, and gives us new insight into the mechanisms by which obese people use food to soothe their emotions," said Dr Wang.

So it's official then – if I'm feeling down I'm going to eat, regardless of whether or not I'm full. And it seems I'm not alone.

A survey by Nimble says that half of British women lie about their dress size and are unable to stick to a diet for more than a couple of days. The study reveals that, because dieting so often ends in failure, women hate admitting to slimming, 63% preferring to say they're 'eating healthily'.

Two-thirds of women are driven to dieting when their clothes feel too tight, and 80% optimistically hang on to clothes that are too small. Around 39% of those surveyed said they avoided fads and preferred to lose weight through a healthy, balanced diet.

Even so, 21% believed they'd be dieting until their 80s. Nutritionist Dr Carrie Ruxton, who has surveyed 50 years of dieting, says it's no wonder that women shy away from revealing their diet habits.

"The word 'diet' these days has negative connotations – it immediately makes us feel set apart and different, and most importantly it raises other people's expectations of us.

"Once you tell people you're on a diet they expect you to look different within a week or a month. If that doesn't happen not only does the person feel a failure inside, but they also feel publicly judged on the outside.

"It has got progressively harder for women," she adds. "In the 50s the hourglass figure was coveted and that was enhanced by wearing corsets and flattering clothes; there was a blip in the 60s with the stick-thin Twiggy era, and then it went into muscled toned bodies like Jane Fonda.

"But nowadays the image is so far off the mark that ordinary women can't come anywhere near it."

Nearly 40% are trying to lose weight, 10% are permanently on a diet, and 20% say they'd like to lose two stone or more. A doctor told me I needed to lose ten. Read that again. TEN.

Wouldn't the thought alone have you reaching for the biscuit tin? I rest my case.

But I refuse to rest on my laurels. Even when they're full…

> # I bought a talking refrigerator that said "Oink" every time I opened the door. It made me hungry for pork chops
>
> ## Marie Mott

WEEK TWO IN BIG Mamma's house and it's all systems go. Yep, my second week of starting Porkers-R-Us online and I'm feeling fine.

In fact, I'm seven pounds lighter according to my mother's bathroom scales – and that wasn't with me doing my normal trick of standing on one leg and squinting so the numbers fade into one.

I don't know what it is about it that seems to be working (legs, arms and other bits crossed) but I think it may have something to do with not allowing myself to overeat. I can indulge, I can stuff my face, I can have whatever I want – but unlike the Atkins where you can have what you like as long as you don't make a sandwich out of it, with the P-R-U, I just can't go over a set-in-stone calorie count.

Me being me, and inhabiting a fantasy land where I feel smaller even after a day of eating sensibly, I decided to treat myself to two things.

The first was a pair of size 20 jeans. I could, of course, have got my inspirational denims from Evans but I wanted to do what 'regular' girls do – I wanted to go out for a weekly shop and throw a pair of jeans in with my fruit (blueberry muffins *do* count apparently) and (not much, granted) veg.

I didn't pay for them, mind you.

Mr Han did, as a little incentive for me to keep plugging away at myself.

(Note to critics: He didn't buy me a size 8 and nor does he really give a stuff if I'm a size 14 or my current 24. I have to believe that or I'll just fade away... but sadly, not by inches).

He cares about my state of mind, not the width of my clothes hangers. But I do see the frustration in his face when we go shopping and he wants to buy me a treat and I end up with a nail file, a candle, make-up or bath stuff.

And that makes him sad.

So, Significant (thin) Other got me jeans and a bra. Yep, a bra.

How many of you normals can just pick up a lovely over-shoulder-boulder-holder with your weekly shop or just pop into M&S for something slinky in your size? Jealous? Moi? You got that right. Anyway, I know what size in clothes I am but bras are another universe because I hate them. There, said it. When I go home after work, the first thing I take off is my bra, as I've said before.

Walking into a regular shop hasn't ever been an option for me, as my measurements are in triple figures and hieroglyphics, apparently.

Instead, it's always been Evans or playing the 'Guess My Size' game for some monstrosity from a free catalogue.

On this occasion we came away with a moulded cup bra (honestly, it looks like a hanging basket without the drainage holes) and something slinky, just because I could.

I'm hoping, though, that in about six months time I'll be using boob tape to take the back in.

Here's hoping for smaller boobs, but slimmer, and yet bigger and better, lingerie ambitions.

What dreadful hot weather we have! It keeps me in a continual state of inelegance

Jane Austen

I CAN'T GO OUT, I can't stay in; I'm hot but covered up in thick clothes and I'm a whisker away from sitting at my desk with my sunglasses on.

Who cares if I look like a freak? All I want to do is hide away from that great globule in the sky that's making me SAD, but the wrong way round.

I have Seasonal Affective Disorder, only in reverse.

I don't hanker for brightness, for sunny days, for heat and light, for short-sleeved shirts, for skirts and flimsy shoes when it is chucking it down outside.

I'm a November baby, built for the comfort of winter – granted, my rainy days are made better for me if shared with people with sunny ways – the whirl of the wind and the crunch of snow beneath my feet. But even alone, it's better cold and wet.

You find less people about during the darker months, invariably dressed in better clothes – there's nobody around pushing their faux cheeriness and G&T tales in your face.

I can 'do' sun, but with conditions, because, and I'm going to be frank here, I simply don't like it.

If truth be told, hot and humid weather makes me nervous.

The amount of people out and about increases, my clothes become inappropriate, headaches become de rigueur, smiles become as fake as Hiya Love's tan in

January, and my underwear becomes restrictive as hell.

Why can't people understand that I'm the living proof that there is no such thing as bad weather, only poor choices in clothing?

Simply put, I loathe the summer. It hangs around me like an ill-fitting suit that makes my legs chafe and arms sweat.

No, give me a rain-soaked early morning, a misty afternoon, a thunderstorm, blizzard and downpour rather than a heat-filled day – any day.

That's the only way you'd be able to turn my twisted SAD into a head full of HAPPY.

Not to mention anything about not being able to dress for summer either. Maybe that's the real reason after all.

> **Carrie: I tried the trapeze yesterday for that piece that I'm writing**
> **Charlotte: I could never! I have the most terrible fear of heights**
> **Carrie: Well, I do not. You've seen my shoes**
>
> *Sex And The City*

SHOES. NOW THERE'S A word that strikes the fear of being fat into me.

I honestly think that I must lack some kind of femininity gene. Because, unlike every other girl I know – with the possible exception of pal Nicola who only does 'sensible' in all aspects of her life – I don't have more than about five pairs of shoes.

When I tell other femmes this, they just look at me with a mixture of sadness and pity on their faces. I read their expression as "Poor cow... fat AND flat soul-ed (sic). Even big girls can look good from the ankle down, chubby chops."

I'm built for comfort and not speed (or even a mild canter, let's be honest), so ease of passage comes above everything else. That means you'll always find me in a pair of sensible flats for work. Oh, and rest. Not forgetting playtime.

I hate shoes. I also hate bras and knickers that look like cheese wire.

When I share the news that I also don't own a matching set of underwear (unless you count mismatched but all black as an outfit) I get the same pitying look as I get regarding shoes.

See what I mean about the girlie gene? I think I got the bad language one instead. I'm 5ft 8ins and I'd love to be knocking 6ft.

So if I could walk on spangly toothpicks with attitude I would tower above most girls. I'd love that look – smug, huge, powerful. Sadly, it would fall flat when I, er, fell flat on my face, stumbling off my perch and into a huge pile of self-negation, then spending about a month wondering why I bothered in the first place.

Besides, who wants to go out in heels, feeling she's so heavy that she runs the risk of going home in flip-flops?

So I stay flat-shoed and comfy, but look longingly at girls who obviously did what I should have done years ago in the privacy of my bedroom while trying to look grown-up – practice.

You know that thing girls do with their mother's shoes? Walking around in big shoes because they want to be a big girl and be able to wear them? I got the big girl part right, but Mam Jones was never into high hells (yes, you read it right) and I was more likely to hanker after a new pair of Paddington Bear red wellies than pom-pom-fronted stilts.

So I was at work the other day and someone was counting how many pairs of shoes they own, while I was busy counting how many calories I'd used up on Porkers-R-Us.

There were so many footwear items on her list, she had to swap a shorthand pad for A4.

Said number-cruncher could name them, visualise them even, while another girl listened intently, wishing she too had as many pairs of toe curlers.

She felt a poor imitation with a measly 25 pairs. Yep, 25 pairs. And no, you're not misreading that. I managed to get to three pairs. Then I remembered my daps. So add one more.

Do slippers count? OK, let's say they do. Boots? Don't count them as they have heels, were a present, and I've never worn them as I don't have a skirt. Besides, last time I was small enough to do the boots/long skirt thing I had bigger hair than I do now and someone told me I looked like Stevie Nicks, which put me right off that look.

Another person piped up that I looked more like Bonnie Tyler.

Enough said. In the end, I got to five pairs of shoes, a number which doesn't tally with the findings of a new survey, which says that women aged over 40 own an average of 19 pairs of shoes, but it is not uncommon to have more than 100. ONE HUNDRED PAIRS OF SHOES.

One hundred more reasons for me to weigh small so I can get seriously tall more like.

Hand on heart, though, I'd love to have a floor full of shoes – high ones, flimsy ones, ridiculously expensive ones, boots, flats, thongs and those that would right the wrongs of my ridiculously limited wardrobe. But there's one big stumbling block – unless they're reinforced with spongy innards (and I'm not talking treacle flavoured either) I can't walk in them.

In my world, the devil not only wears Prada. She tops it off with a high pair of bottoms.

THE ODDEST THINGS WILL set me off 'on one', sliding downwards into a pit of jumbled thinking until I land – splat! – face-down in the pile of nonsensical gunk that is my self-esteem (or lack thereof).

For a fortnight I'd been feeling fine, meaning I'd been tottering around like a footballer's wife in an expensive pair of toothpicks, thinking that even if I didn't have it going on I was doing just fine.

I even went for four long walks with my friend Justin, cut my croissant intake down to one at the weekend instead of six (that's stretched over three days, mind you), tried to slice out sliced bread and generally be good and healthy. I even did a few miles on the exercise bike.

So all was going well until I started thinking I had no business being in fantasy footwear at all.

And that's because someone I met made me – unwittingly so, I have to say – feel like a fairy camel next to her.

This, coupled with the fact that I had to have some new photographs taken, landed me in a right old mood.

Let's take the photo fiasco first. Significant (thin) Other is a film editor, and as a side-line he takes pictures, mostly of the spaces normal-eyed people wouldn't even give passing consideration to.

But in a moment of madness, he asked to take some portraits of me. So there I was, big-eyed and feeling

149

confident, posing and preening, thinking I was finally going to see something nice in these pictures, that he was going to unearth similarly fascinating and previously unseen spaces in my genetic make-up.

It lasted all of two minutes – until I saw the snaps.

I can only describe my reaction as stupid, but it was my kind of stupid.

I looked fat-faced. Fat of face. Fat in the face. Fat. And I cried. It was behind my eyes, so that he wouldn't see, but I felt, at that moment, that another dent in my already shaky armour had been made.

I went home from my photo shoot (a glamorous way of saying he stuck a white sheet up behind my head in his bathroom) gutted, with all the usual self-negating stuff flying around in my noodle.

How did I get to this? Where did it all go wrong? Why can't I see anything attractive when I look at myself? Why, you silly cow, weren't you satisfied at a size 18, 20 or even a 22? Why do you put yourself through this idiocy every single day?

Of course I got over it – but it took a three-hour drive, lots of "oohing" and "aaaahing" and "you're fabulousing" from my special snapper, platitudes from Hiya Love and my mother going "they're lovely, 'Anna – do you think he'll print a few up for me?"

And me? Well, I'm still not convinced.

But I am certain, however, that I'm not the best person to judge the value of me.

It's not my job, but I wish it were. Then I would have all the tools at my disposal to think that I am – and look – great, no matter what.

This would have helped me out greatly with issue number two – the wedding planner.

Don't worry, I'm not getting hitched (do NOT get me

started on what I'd wear in my make believe wedding please) but I had to meet the wedding planner for a story I was doing.

I went downstairs at work to greet her and I was assaulted by a vision of understated elegance in polkadots.

I had on clumpy, sensible springer shoes; she wore dainty pointy things, emblazoned with a different type of spot to her wraparound top. She carried her portfolio and huge white bag like a New York wife, balancing the day's work with the kind of grace you can't buy on sale at Evans.

And there I was, as graceful as being caught with beef dripping running down my fingers on a Sunday lunchtime, thinking I'd never, *ever* be a Laura Ashley wife or so goldarn pleasant to boot.

And that's because I think I'm too busy being – oh dear, I can't believe I'm even going to say this word now – average.

There was a time when I didn't think I was the 'A' word, but my sense of fabulousness would always take a battering as soon as someone said, in the varying stages of weight gain, "You're nice-looking, isn't it a shame you're fat."

If only I'd stopped hearing these voices at size 18, I'd be less fragmented about my sense of self now. So the wedding planner left me smiling, laughing, and sending me an email saying she had a fabulous time in my company. I put that through my Hannah Filter and it came out as, "You're great! It's right what they say about hanging out with people fatter than you, it makes you look smaller. Thanks *so much* for that!"

Seriously though, I know she laughed and I know she smiled. So did I, but it was only after she'd gone and, two days later, as I made my way breathlessly up the stairs (I'm so good, I've not taken the lift at work once in three weeks now), that I realised that high heels don't make the woman, and neither do petite shoulders.

But I admit it – I'd sell my soul for just one day of feeling feminine and upbeat about my body and my face.

Not to mention having a picture taken while looking simply stunning in polka-dots.

> **People say that losing weight is no walk in the park. When I hear that I think, yeah, that's the problem**
>
> **Chris Adams**

DOES A CAN OF Sugar-Free So Your Life Tastes Sweeter pop somehow negate a corned beef and onion baguette?

I didn't have butter on it, there were no sauces or pickle in sight. So I've just this second told myself that I was being a good girl and as such, I've topped off my lunch with a low-cal muffin and, for extra food group goodness, a chocolate-covered flapjack.

It was only recently, though, that I realised that even good food is bad for you.

Years ago, a family friend was trying a certain well known diet yet again.

"You should go on it," she enthused, before she fell off the wagon and into a vat of beef curry (with boiled rice, for good measure).

"You can eat all the chicken you want; you can cook a whole one a day and nibble on it. Hey, you can cook 12 a day and nibble on them! You won't put on any weight."

It was good news for this limited variety foodie, until I realised that I couldn't eat anything with the chicken and you could get fowl pest from being a dietary pest.

The All You Can Eat promise appealed to me, Miss Can't Moderate Anything, until someone with enough medical certificates to paper a small bungalow told me years later, "Yes, there are such things as good foods but remember, if you fill up on just good foods you're still

153

taking in loads of calories."

And the funny thing is, I didn't even realise this.

I thought, in my calorie-uncontrolled ignorance, that I could just stuff myself with fat-free nonsense and sugar substitute goodies until the smug and svelte cows came home. Not so.

The same (formerly fat) medicine man also told me that losing two pounds a week wasn't good enough (as if I wasn't depressed already). When I complained that I WAS eating sensibly and that I WAS doing eight miles a night on my exercise bike which took me around half an hour, he looked me straight in the eye and said, "Not good enough, my girl. You need to do an hour at least."

So what's a girl to do?

Simple, convince myself somehow that just talking about doing it, isn't actually leading the good life.

On my twice-weekly walk with Justin last week – 40 minutes of absolute calf-splitting hell, I may add – we spent the time musing on the diets we have both loved (i.e. hated) and lost (not a lot of weight on).

Both of us, officially serial dieters, found that we'd lost the most weight on diets where you don't have to moderate certain foods, but are obliged, on pain of clogged arteries, to cut out others.

I lost about three stone on the Atkins – the diet where you can eat what you like, as long as you don't make a pasta salad or torpedo roll out of it.

For Justin, it was eating six small meals a day and only cutting out sugar. And on a Sunday, the day when the good Lord rested, Justin also took a break, but it was from the diet.

Instead he sprang into chewing action as he was positively encouraged to indulge in 'bad' food until he was bursting.

So Sunday became his Sinday, where he was able to eat his body weight in McDonald's, pizza, chips and all the inch nudging stuff 'ordinary' folk indulge in now and again.

He also went to the gym six times a week; on my successful stint I got myself a treadmill and did a little bit of fast walking in my bedroom. And here's a fast fat fact for you – we're both right back at the place where we started from.

And that is fat, certainly bigger than before our lifetime of new beginnings on diets.

Of course we both joke that we're as hilarious as ever, as gorgeous as ever, as brilliant as ever, and as delusional as ever. But the only thing we don't really laugh at is knowing there's something in us both that doesn't enable us to stay at a certain weight and be happy about it.

At least we have each other to sigh with.

And that *can* be more fulfilling than strawberry cheesecake while you're waiting for a Chinese to be delivered.

> **I'm not fanatical. I've learned how to deal with diets. My muscles have memory from the time I danced, and it's quick for me to get back in shape. But I'm not fanatical**
>
> **Catherine Zeta-Jones**

NOTHING MUCH HAS HAPPENED this week, but there have been some lowlights.

For some reason, they all happened on Wednesday.

First of all I exceeded my allowance on the Porkers-R-Us diet with aplomb.

Then someone at work brought cakes in. I resisted for three hours – three hours! – but gave up in the end.

Next up I had two (just the two, mind) pieces of pizza, avoided a chocolate muffin but ate my body weight (considerable) in dips (low fat) and chips (sans salt).

I also discovered on said Wednesday that I'm too fat to go into the Army.

No surprise there, perhaps, and definitely less than when I found out that, even with a good degree in Philosophy, I couldn't train as a teacher as I had three Es and an F in maths (the last one with a year's private tuition thrown in).

A girl can resign herself to lots of things, and in the great tapestry of life's chips'n'dips, much of it can be rationalised.

No, the real downer came when I discovered my richer, more beautiful, classier, far-more-talented-but-can't-hold-down-a-proper-Welsh-accent-to-save-her-life namesake is on the same diet at me.

Yes, Catherine Zeta-Jones has apparently dropped from a 'whopping' (hold me back) size 14 to a 'fabulously sexy' size 10.

'Zeta-Bones' was pictured at an awards ceremony in New York looking slinky in a designer dress by Tory Burch (I had to look that bit up) with stillies from Roger Vivier (who?).

Anyway, 'Less-Eater Jones' (I should be working for The Mirror not spending my time looking in one and wanting to smash the bugger) has always been big (oh, they just keep on coming, don't they?) on glamour and has never succumbed to that size zero fetish, so prevalent with starlets, to be smaller than their shoe size.

Always described as 'curvy' by headline writers who obviously have never been to an all-you-can-eat carvery in a Valleys pub, she was reported as saying that she's followed a sensible eating plan to shed some extra pounds.

Where she was hiding her extra poundage is anyone's guess, though. I can only assume it was in her deep pockets.

Anyway, 'Sleeka-Jones' (OK, I'll stop now) still has a bit of meat on her bones, albeit not a lot to feed a starving dog on. She has, however, stored up enough common sense to have a refreshing attitude to dieting. She said, "Sure, I have to watch what I eat to stay in shape. We all do.

"But I'm not fanatical. I've learned how to deal with diets."

As if a sensible attitude to losing weight wasn't enough, the lucky cow added, "My muscles have memory from the time I danced, and it's quick for me to get back in shape. But I'm not fanatical."

The only memory my muscles have is of the one time

I took the stairs instead of the lift. Yep, it's still a painful one for the soft sods.

Our Cath, who is now in the running for a medal the size of a non-stick frying pan for services to dietary nous, has also had a go in the past at some actresses for rushing to shed post-pregnancy weight so they can meet Hollywood's demand for stick-thin leading ladies. She went as far as calling them "insane".

The actress, who has two young children with Michael Douglas, contrasted her own steady return to her 'normal' figure with the trend some celebs are setting of 'competing' to get back to their usual weight as soon as possible.

"I grew up with dancers – anorexia and other eating disorders were common – so I learned how to deal with diets without losing my limit.

"I think it's awful, this competition between actresses who've just had a baby to see who's first to get back to their normal weight. It's insane. I find this wave of super-skinny women scary," she's reported as saying in the newspapers today.

I guess, then, that she doesn't think a size 10 is super-skinny.

I had this argument with people at work the other day.

I was bleating on about the fact that I don't consider a size 10 to be necessarily 'curvy'; and the thinnies disagreed.

Well they would, wouldn't they? I said size 10 girls can be shapely, but that the word 'curvy' was perhaps best left to women sized 16-plus, or 14, at a push.

Girls who go seriously in, and seriously out, so they can seriously shake it all about. No, they said – just look at Katherine Jenkins. The singer is also a size 10 and, I have to admit, very shapely.

But curvy? Sure, she has a great boobs/waist/hips ratio. But she doesn't really have any excess stuff to shimmy all about, does she?

To me, she's slim with a twist, a girl who can't pinch more than an inch but who has an hour-glass silhouette. Petite perfection, some would say. Unlike CZ-J, Kath has always been tiny, always been small – not that I would ever call 'Zeta Lost Stones' (sorry, couldn't resist it) large. No, what I can't quite get my head around is why less is more... even when you're less than a size 16 to start with.

I'M FEELING ALL FRACTIOUS. I've just had some crushing news and I don't know what to do with myself. Like a boozer seeking comfort and clarification at the bottom of a glass, I'm debating whether to cheese and onion my sorrows away with a packet of crisps. No big deal, you might think, but when I use food to ease my mood, I start thinking I'm back on the slippery slope of defeatism.

So, I know crisps would just be the start of it. I'd get a taste for them and I'd have another packet.

Then I'd convince myself that, having been a good girl over the past few weeks, a bar of something chocolaty from the sweets machine at work would be fine.

Or a truck-sized Yorkie. Or lunch-time sandwiches eaten for breakfast. When I'm thinking straight, none of this matters and I don't overeat in a dream-like daze of indifference.

But Mondays are weigh-days.

They're also, for serial body-battlers like me, make or break days. And I've been good, been as focused as I get.

Only this week, I find I've stayed exactly the same weight as last week. And I have the certificate to prove it, burning a hole in the pocket of my new size 22 (read that again) winter coat.

I'm antsy, itching to indulge because I'm disappointed in myself and that's what I normally do when I feel like this. I emotionally stuff myself. I emotionally starve myself, too. I can multi-task, me.

So what to do? How do I put a stop to the endless not-so-merry-go-round of feeling enthused then deflated, the point at which I start eating for Wales?

According to agony aunt Jenni Trent-Hughes at www.slimhappy.co.uk (that's an oxymoron if ever I heard one), goal setting is the way to go.

She says, "How do we get happy about what we're doing, make it all visible immediately and get results from day one? We score ourselves. Establish what we want to accomplish and keep track of it. Every time we put a check in a box say, "well done that woman!

"Here's the secret to setting 'good' goals – you cannot control how much weight you lose. But you can control what efforts you take to lose it, so that's what you base your goals on. Your goal isn't 'lose two pounds in the first week' – you may and, then again, you may not.

"Your goal is 'Walk for 20 minutes today'. 'Go through the day without eating a biscuit' – check. If you set these goals correctly you'll soon find 'Lose lots of weight' will happen before you know it."

So how do you score disappointment, then?

Simple, says Jenni – you just stay away from the scales.

"This is the hardest one for some of us to stick to, but I have to say that I've been doing it now for six weeks (only weighed myself twice) and I now understand the experts who swear by it.

"If you're in an organised programme they want you to weigh once a week but, if you're doing this on your own, or with us here, there's no real need for that.

"The woman who started me out on this journey advises once a month, three days after your period ends.

For this whole project to work, especially if you've got a lot of weight to shift, you need to take the focus past the numbers and put it onto a shiny new you."

That's all well and good but mere mortals like me have to see results in order to know we're on the right track. I don't know about you but I'm not woman enough to just BELIEVE I'm doing well or have the patience to wait for the once-a-month ritual.

But maybe there is something in it. Maybe the trick is, as Jenni tells me, just to be happy with who you are. The rest, she promises, will follow.

"Get a piece of paper and write down five things about yourself that you or others in your life really like about you," she advises. "Read it out loud twice. 'I am fun to be with', 'I am good at sudoku' – whatever.

"How do you feel? Chances are you're smiling.

"You may have a few more pounds than you want. You may be worried about how you're going to fit into your Granny's old wedding frock but the fact of the matter is there are a few good things about you already in place. Learn to value them more than you probably do now. Stop thinking of yourself as someone who needs to lose weight first and foremost.

"That is not who you are. Yes, that is part of you but it's number six, focus on numbers one, two, three, four, five!"

The trouble is, I'm shit at figures. But a dab hand at slating my own.

Beauty is only skin deep, but ugly goes clean to the bone

Dorothy Parker

I NEARLY CRIED. I admit I did sigh. Then I started feeling ridiculously out of place and disenchanted.

It was supposed to be a treat, meant to relax me, pamper me, and leave me feeling like the living/walking/talking/breathing embodiment of a Carpenters song.

But, as soon as I walked into the spa (not one of those that sells pasties that you can warm up while you wait either) and was handed a terry-towelling bundle, I knew I would find myself a long way off feeling on top of the world and looking down on creation.

Half and hour early for my 105-minute session, I sat fully clothed in the 'Relaxation Room' waiting for my treatment to begin.

Only a pair of white slippers differentiated me from the lunch crowd, like I was there to do a VAT inspection in comfort, rather than partake of a health kick (this one right up my arse).

A big fluffy white robe and a beauty uniform that sat bunched up in a ball on the sun lounger beside me, unused, is not something I'd wear

As soon as the lady in reception handed it to me, images of a previous bad spa experience came crowding in. And why? Because I knew it wouldn't fit me.

Trying to show willing, I quickly took my stash, locked myself in a cubicle and tried it on, just in case.

It fitted – as long as I didn't do it up. I also looked like the Michelin Man gone wrong.

It was a one-size-fits-all embarrassment that left me frustrated and annoyed that spas, even the nicest and most well-intentioned, don't cater for people like me.

All I could do was walk up the stairs to the RR, plonk my fully clothed but fluffy-feeted fat arse on the lounger and try to look inconspicuous as other people waltzed in and out – all in perfectly fitting dressing gowns.

I sat there, feeling like a right old lump of lard, and mused on the last time I had experienced such humiliation – perhaps it was the time 90201 was a show and not how many pounds I imagined I weighed.

Then as now, I'd gone to a five-star facility and was given a white robe to deck myself out in.

Then, as now, I'd gone dutifully to change out of my clothes and walk around like a half-baked Hollywood wife while I waited to be 'treated'.

But, of course, it didn't touch me. Hmpf. Time for plan B, I thought.

Off I trundled to the swanky reception area, to ask if they happened to have one in a larger size.

This is the conversation that ensued.

Nasty cow: *"Is everything all right, Miss Jones? Why aren't you changed? Your treatment is about to begin...."*

Me: *"Yeah, ummm, sorry. The robe doesn't fit me. Do you have a bigger one, please?"*

Nasty cow: *"Doesn't fit? Surely not – our robes are massive... "*

Me (trying to keep the volume down and stop myself from grabbing her by the throat): *"It doesn't fit. I need a bigger one. Sorry for the inconvenience."*

Nasty cow: *"Have you tried pulling it tighter?"*

Me: *"Well, yes, I suppose so. But as it's really thick, I don't think it will go much tighter. There's no give, see. It doesn't fit, see. So, so sorry."*

Nasty cow: *"These robes, madam, are made to fit ANYONE. I suppose I could go and see if we have any in the men's spa but I doubt they'd have* your *size there anyway. They really are quite roomy, you know. Oh well, you'll just have to wear your own clothes then. But we can't be responsible for them. Do the slippers fit at least or do you need a* special *pair of those?"*

Me: *"Shut up, you over-stuffed, plastic-looking, ignorant bitch. You know what? I can lose my weight but you're going to be stuck with that fucking ugly face for ever!"*

I made that last bit up, but honestly, I was stunned by the insensitivity of it all.

Luckily though, on this occasion things were different, despite the similarity of ill-fitting bathrobes.

Lovely therapist Natasha, booked to give me a Tuck & Suck It Up treatment (based on Chinese massage and the Russian School of massage principles and incorporating products and snore-inducing blissful massage for double-action slimming and firming) couldn't have been nicer.

Before she could get a word out, I told her the robe wouldn't fit me and, bless her 5ft, size 8 heart, she simply said, "Loads of people can't fit into them. Don't worry about it – you won't need it. As long as you feel OK, we'll be fine. Now, let me tell you about your treatment today."

From then on, spirits slightly lifted but feeling awkward as she asked me what parts of my body I thought needed slimming or toning up – I bit my tongue and stopped myself from saying, "Haven't you got eyes in your pretty little head, sweet lips?" – I settled back to enjoy it.

Honestly, it was fabulous – and although I can't see it's made any difference to the way I look, it was a luxurious experience as I was wrapped up in cling-film, plastered with what looked like chocolate icing, and left to sink into a dreamy state while it set

She even massaged my belly – if anyone is putting together nominations for OBEs, please take note.

At £95, the treatment wasn't cheap, and luckily I was having it gratis so I could review it for 'work'.

But I think it's worth the price for knowing that even the tiniest of people sometimes don't think you're a freak just because you can't wear white.

> **This guy says, 'I'm perfect for you, because
> I'm a cross between a macho
> and a sensitive man.'
> I said, 'Oh, a gay trucker?'**
>
> **Judy Tenuta**

I'VE BEEN REALLY GOOD lately. For three weeks I've eaten low fat, my portions have been smaller and I've been doing 20 minutes of sweat-inducing activity on my exercise bike every other night.

OK, I admit that I haven't been doing it at weekends, but I don't want the present Mr Han seeing me sweat like a bullock.

The late Paula Yates, during happier times with Bob Geldof, said that one of the secrets to their then happy marriage was that he didn't see her doing girlie things like shaving her legs and underarms, colouring her hair etc.

She would just appear before him like a femme fatale, like she had just stepped out of a salon.

Luckily for me, I'm fair and don't need to shave – my family jokes that I'm the only person in the world with blonde roots – but I like to keep a bit of mystery, too.

Like Paula, I like to maintain a semblance of dignity and not show him that I can't pedal for more than a minute without looking like I've run a full marathon. Naked.

Anyway, feeling that my clothes were looser and that my double chin was starting to disappear, I decided to pop on the scales in Boots and imagine myself looking in wonder as the numbers melted away like chip fat in a frying pan.

I was expecting at least an eight-pound reduction after all my hard work. And I was really, really surprised by what I saw.

No, not that I'd lost nine pounds or even a stone. I'd put on point two of a kilogram.

Read that again – three weeks of dieting and exercise and I'd put on weight.

How the hell did that happen?

I'd been good, halo-inducing good, and it's been for nothing.

Depressed, disappointed and angry at myself, I got home and had Chicken Kiev (two; healthy eating ones) and chips (loads; chunky ones, so there was less fat).

Eating bad (but I'd only really had about 500 calories tops that day) was my personal platinum plated punishment for not losing a pound.

Hiya Love – who topped off his lot with grated cheese and beans – tried to convince me that I was eating 'sensibly' and I deserved a reward.

I wasn't convinced, and although I haven't cheated big-style since then, I'm finding it hard not to rush over to Boots and take advantage with my Advantage Card on their 3-4-1 deal on Shapers crisps and snacks.

I did it the other day in fact, and promptly ate the lot within the hour. I added up my total at the end of the day and, even with the meal deal, I'd not reached the recommended 1,200 calories.

At least I've been trying to treat myself better. Yeah, so it's not done me any good on the scales, but I'm making every effort to be a better me.

My problem is I get tired, too easily, of the amount of effort it takes to be good. It also tries my patience like nothing else on earth.

The other day, for example, I took a phone call from a personal trainer in Barry who called me a "lovely looking girl" who "needs to get real" with herself.

For a few moments, he talked at me about aims, goals, ambitions and something about us running the London Marathon.

He said he'd "love to work" with me, and that he'd get me fit and healthy, and "back on track".

Men, eh? They're full of false promises. Not that I doubt that he is a fine trainer, but in the words of every other woman I've known, I've heard it all before.

Besides, I just don't get upbeat 'people power' as I'm not like it myself.

I'm a defeatist before I start – so it's not easy being 'up' for the challenge when someone fitter than me demands that I be as self-believing in my capabilities as they are in their own taut-muscled bodies.

This kind of Yankee babble just frustrates me and renders me speechless.

People who say "you can't want it bad enough then"… well, you have absolutely no idea what it's like to be trapped by your own limitations. But hey, I know mine and I make no excuses for them – just don't ask me to change my reality on ideologies I could read off the back of a cereal packet.

That said, I've had a few personal trainers in my time and they've all been fabulous, all been patient, and all at least tried to be sympathetic in that tough-love kind of way.

But despite their strengths, wash-board stomachs and 'you can do this!' cajoling, they all failed with me.

Big Bugger was the first.

A skinhead with a Freddie Mercury fetish, he helped

me lose a few stone and got me to run. Run! And I don't just mean to Burger King when the bacon double cheeseburgers are on offer.

The first time we – and I credit him with this – achieved it, it was like someone had given me a million pounds.

I felt normal, I felt alive, I felt capable of all kinds of silly little things for the first time in years. But then I moved house – going to see him was geographically impossible – and my finances changed, so BB fell by the wayside as did my resolve.

Next up was Abs. God, how I adored Abs.

He had a 'big' girlfriend, a heart of gold, and could talk for Wales in a Scottish accent.

He knew I hated the gym, so we'd go boxing instead; he suggested little life changes to me like walking up a flight of stairs to go to the toilet on another floor; but more than that, he made me think I could move mountains with my mind.

Then my working situation changed and I couldn't get to him during sensible hours.

So he left my life kicking and screaming, while I said goodbye with a small backwards wave, relieved I wasn't obliged to feel hot and certainly bothered anymore.

Having a trainer was an extreme act for me, and I don't think I'm ready to do it again. Not that I'm a commitment-phobe, but as I said earlier I just don't like looking like shit in front of well-toned and upbeat people, as well as feeling like it.

So I'll keep on plugging away – just me, my exercise bike, and food served on a tea plate.

With my bedmate Frustration for company.

> **The gods had condemned Sisyphus to ceaselessly rolling a rock to the top of a mountain, whence the stone would fall back of its own weight. They had thought with some reason that there is no more dreadful punishment than futile and hopeless labour**
>
> **Albert Camus**

THINGS ON MY MIND, part 99.

1. Significant (thin) Other is moving in. That means I can't hang around the house bra-less in case he thinks my breasts have morphed into Jubblies that aren't so lovely. I can't hide food either – he's far too savvy for that. Or walk around half-naked. Or be constantly miserable about the way I look. He can put up with weekend bouts of the blues, but my daily dressing-downs of myself are not conducive to a harmonious love nest, I'm sure.

2. I'm 35 on Sunday.

3. As a result of thinking I will use that day to mark yet another First Day of the Rest of My Life and finally either accept me for me or try harder to be a smaller, fitter version of me, I'm eating for Wales.

4. Today's menu: nothing for breakfast. So I congratulate myself with a ham roll, packet of crisps, two biscuits and a cheese and onion pasty. I'm fancying a fresh cream

apple turnover now. Funny how I NEVER want to indulge like this when I'm not on a diet. If only I had the brains to follow the logic then stick to it once it's settled in my thick skull.

5. My bra feels tight. And it's a new one. Surely I couldn't have gone from 42G (Jesus Christ!) to 89ZZ overnight? I feel fat. Hey, I look fat. At least my boobs are buoyant. Quite unlike my mood.

6. Someone put a cutting from a magazine on my desk. The top tip for losing weight was a stupid, 'Try wearing a fancy bracelet on the hand you hold your fork in – it'll remind you of how much you're eating.' Whatever next? Carrying a pair of size 14 jeans in my bag, a pound of lard in my pocket or a picture of a pig in my purse? I can only oink at the fuzzy logic of it all.

7. As of Thursday, my mother's lost three stone. Why didn't I inherit her resolve gene?

8. Do I look like Hattie Jacques?

9. Hmmm, would it matter if I did? Someone at work heard me musing on this and said I reminded them more of Bernard Manning. Yes, THAT Bernard Manning. And I don't think he meant that I was hilarious.

10. I met a girl who's going to have a gastric bypass. She's just one stone heavier than me and one clothes size bigger. She has a few more chins, but who am I to judge? I was jealous. We went to see the same bloke at Morriston Hospital in Swansea. He said I didn't look "what" I am (i.e. weight etc) and that I didn't need

surgery. Just "try a bit harder" on my own. The bloke was a comic with a sideline in amassing medical certificates. The worst kind. The other girl did, apparently, look clinically obese (nice, eh?) enough to warrant the surgery.

When I told her I'd been turned down, maybe she thought I was wearing a fancy bracelet on my fork-holding hand which, when I pinged it, enable me to lie about my vital statistics.

I'm prepared to show my wrists and take a lie detector test when I meet her next.

11. I need to get my fringe cut, but I can't bear the thought of being plonked in front of a mirror and coming out with flat hair. A girl needs volume like she needs air. Bend me, shake me, move me anyway you want me – as long as I'll come out big haired, that's all right.

12. What if S(thin)O wants children? Can they do ultrasounds over a fat belly?

13. I thought uber-skinny girl Marianne from Channel 5's *Make Me A Supermodel* was nicer-looking than the 'curvier' (pa'leeese!) size 12, gobby Jen. Mind you, neither was any great shakes. Marianne was a shapeless albeit stunning, stick; Jen had a family-sized muffin top over her jeans and gnat bites for boobs. I seem to have elephant chunks.

14. S(thin)O tells me via text that I'm gorgeous and the perfect person to spend his life with. I don't need to laminate the message to believe it, but I don't think I can hear violins. I can just about make out the harmonics of hope and acceptance, though.

15. But it's being drowned out by the voice in my head which is wondering if bangles are on offer in Accessorize today.

> **Think like a queen. A queen is not afraid to fail. Failure is another stepping stone to greatness**
>
> **Oprah Winfrey**

I'M NOT SCARED OF much, but there are a few things that trouble me.

Fish, and wet food collected at the bottom of the sink are two that spring to mind. Oh, and the smell of bins. Oddities, maybe – but they make me baulk.

What really scares me to death is the thought of having to dress in a body suit. I could brave heights, swim under glass and jump out of a plane à la *I'm A Celebrity... Get Me Out Of Here!*

But the thought of being picked to do a challenge and having to do it wearing a yellow jump-suit is enough to make me heave.

When Jan Leeming and that awful Scott Whatshischops did that thing where he had to dangle midair on a rope ladder and throw balloons for her to catch while balancing on a tightrope, I was almost in tears.

And that's because, at that very moment, the colour of my perceived self-imposed limitations slapped me in the face.

I imagined myself in the jungle, and the fear of having to wear shorts, a bra top and khaki-coloured what-nots was palpable.

There I was, sat on the settee thinking that nothing out

there would be too big to handle, that I'd be able to show the world how dexterous I am, how able, how gutsy – for a lumper like me (see, always making allowances for myself because of my dress size).

When Jan and Whinger came on looking like Caped Custard Crusaders, I knew that if I had been set that challenge I would have said no problem; if I had then been shown what I would have to wear, I would have chickened it. No question at all. In a heartbeat. No discussion needed.

Odd, isn't it, to be limited by your body and what you think other people will say about it?

To think you're capable of anything – unless you have to show the world you can do it while wearing a skin-hugging sheath. I'm not one of those loud and proud biggies who just gets on with stuff, who doesn't give a bugger what they look like, who goes around saying life's too short to worry and all that greeting card nonsense.

I care too much about my state of mind to not worry about other people's misconceptions of me.

The fact is, I don't want to parade my belly around or celebrate my love handles.

My thighs would stop a pig in a passage and the tops of my arms are so big I could wave them about in the garden and power up the whole street for a year.

To me, my double chins don't necessarily mean double the fun. That said, I don't feel incapable of leading a normal life; doing things that other girls do. I just choose not to do it while looking stupid. Or jogging.

I wish I were smaller, but I'm not; I wish I could see that I'm not bad-looking, but I can't; I'd love to accept me as I am and embrace the plus (no pun intended) points of my character. Fat fucking chance.

But I'll tell you something for nothing – it would have taken more than a fear of heights, snakes or crocs to hold me back from the balloon challenge. And that's not because there was the promise of food at the end of it.

No, I would have gone in with all Valleys' girl chutzpah blazing – but only if I was allowed to do it in wide-legged trousers and a nice smock top as part of the deal.

Ice cream is happiness condensed

Jessi Lane Adams

DID YOU KNOW THERE'S an Organisation for Lesbians of Size? Well now you do.

I've recently discovered a network for size 'self-esteem', the Plus USA Woman Pageant and Convention, more2hug.com, Life in the Fat Lane blogger and the site Imabiggal.com. I also found out that a national music magazine supposedly pulled a front page featuring singing 'fat activist' Beth Ditto because she's, well, not shaped like Cerys Matthews. And she likes to strip off and show the world her, er, charms. Beats me how anyone would want to run around semi-naked, inches pinching, for all the world to see.

But neither bravery nor a couldn't-give-a-shit attitude are my strongest points.

Then I heard Joanna Lumley had initially been turned down as a model because she was 'too fat, too ugly' and that Nigella Lawson has never met a doughnut she didn't like. Neither have I... or a pizza, Yorkshire pudding or bakery, come to think of it.

Nige says of her body image, "We're all worrying endlessly, it's relaxing to think I don't have to fight the fight any more, life is so much rosier."

She could say that, of course, with a face like that and certified domestic goddess status.

I imagine she's the kind of woman who would get away with NOT inviting someone over for dinner just because her grandmamma didn't bother, and she's a traditional sort.

And people, in that schmoozy way they do with the talented/good-looking/posh lot, would simply smile and think it marvellously eccentric of her.

But you've got to have money to be eccentric – poor fat folk like me would simply sound crackers. So where did all this information come from?

Do you imagine me sitting around surfing the web, reading magazines, watching the telly looking for fatbits – you know, like titbits but with more in the arse department. If so, you would be wrong. Because what with being the token biggie in the office, and writing this column – I mean, how many times can I say I'm big and wish I wasn't, in 1,000 words? – comes people's interest in all things related to size.

So colleagues leave articles on my desk and email me news about who's said what and who's wearing what; diet tips, press releases on appetite suppressants, gym opening times and the odd (really bloody odd) list of positive affirmations. Because, as someone reminded me this week, with the aid of a Whitney Houston ring-tone, the greatest love of all is inside of me.

And then there came this week's piece de resistance – a newspaper cutting of Vanessa Feltz with the words, written, AND THEN HIGHLIGHTED, across it by an anonymous supporter, "You're nicer-looking than her. What size do you think she is? Bigger than you I bet."

Smaller than me more like, came my silent response to my mystery friend.

La Feltz, who is doing the rounds banging on about her new TV show, has never been backwards in coming forwards about stuff, as she has opinions on opinions.

She's also remained remarkably upbeat despite her very public marriage split, and some, less cynical than me, would say the woman-scorned role has somewhat bolstered her career.

As a role model for bigger ladies, she's not a bad one. Of course she's lost weight – she went from a size 26 to a 12 with the help of personal trainer turned lover. Then she made a fitness/lifestyle video.

I know 'cos I bought it thinking that if a fellow biggie can do it, so could I (wrong). And after that she did what fellow battlers do – she put some of it back on, but still managed to remain philosophical about it.

These days she looks, to my untrained eye, about a size 18-20. But her size isn't what comes immediately to my mind – why should it, right?

I think of her and what comes to my mind is a gobby, confident, bright, unnecessarily spangly (clothes wise), someone who dresses at least 10 years too young, earnest, wise, too brassy-blonde and long-haired for her age. And amidst my smorgasbord of responses is also empathy.

Because she, for all her Cambridge-educated ramblings, brain-box power and success, still finds it difficult to cope with the constant attention to her weight. Join the club, Fuzzy Feltz.

"It's always in the papers," she says. "I remember having lunch with an old school friend and someone phoned my lawyer and said 'We've got the sushi pictures', and so he phoned me and I was like 'What was I doing? Inhaling it?'," she says in an interview today, with a self-deprecating laugh.

"Honestly, it's ridiculous. I once bought a pair of knickers in a size 18 and even that made the papers."

Vanessa freely admits that her size isn't something that she has been afraid to talk publicly about – she's made an appearance in *Little Britain*'s Fat Fighters

180

sketch and taken part in the second series of *Celebrity Fit Club*.

But she says it's a step too far when strangers make hurtful comments to her face. "The sorts of things that people's mothers or husbands might say to them once every 10 years like 'perhaps you shouldn't eat that pie', total strangers say to me almost every minute of every day.

"People feel that it's part of a common currency to discuss my weight – I am used to it after all these years but it's not great for me, I don't love it."

And therein lies a lesson to all of you well-intentioned lovelies who try to support us plus-size moaners. Hear us out when we're blue about the big battle of the bulge, just don't berate us for wanting to be more self-accepting but not quite managing it; know that we DO take responsibility for being as we are, but please never EVER tell us to put that pie down.

Life in the large lane isn't all about pastry, you know. It is, however, about being a flawed and massively sensitive human being…

OK, and one whose idea of moderation is only knowing how to spell it.

A waist is a terrible thing to mind

Tom Wilson

HERE'S A CHRISTMAS MIRACLE for you. Well, it's not so much a miracle as a piece of advice – if you follow it, though, it will be like the second coming.

Christmas decorations can be glittery and over the top – YOUR CLOTHES CAN'T!

Do not make the mistake of losing your mind at Christmas time. It's not an excuse to look like a giant bauble with facial hair; it's a time to delicately go about your business and keep a cool head while other less curvy girls are losing theirs in strapless over-the-shoulder-boulder-holders (sigh) and shiny tops. In truth, I don't generally go to Christmas parties. But I have got one coming up soon which, as ever, has got me in a right state about what to wear.

Black trousers and a black top won't quite cut it. So what do you do to snazzy things up a bit, while being careful not to run the risk of looking like a Christmas pudding?

If you can afford it, have a look at www.box2.co.uk There's a store in Bristol and at the Capitol Centre in Cardiff. We're talking jackets at £130 and trousers about £40. But the clothes are wonderfully swishy, original and just the right side of arty – stylish, but not outlandish.

If money's a little tighter, Evans is your best bet. But I have to say I've been largely unimpressed with their stock this year. Halter-neck tops in satin, pom-pom skirts and calf-length, strapless dresses aren't a good look on us

182

zaftig goddesses (yeah, I'm in a good mood today).

So be sure you don't just pick up something which'll make you look like a turkey without the stuffing, just because you've got a do to go to.

Trust me, you'll look a million times better in something less 'of the moment' (NEVER follow a trend girls, especially if it comes in gold, with a drop waist, cut-off tights and pea-sized clutch bag) than trussed up like your thin counterparts.

Think about this – you'll want to look good when first in line at the buffet, so you don't want to stand out for looking anything less than stunning, do you?

> **The older you get, the tougher it is to lose weight, because by then your body and your fat are really good friends**
>
> **Anonymous**

HERE'S A QUESTION MY mother never needed to answer. Would she have opted for me to have surgery because I was a plump child?

Say I was a nine-year-old fatty and the NHS had the power to perform a little nip and tuck on not-so-littles like me, would she have said that I could have had it done?

To be honest, I don't think she would have even given that suggestion head room – then again, she, along with the rest of my family, did think I'd lose my 'puppy fat' when I was 16.

Sixteen came, as did 26, and 36 will come knocking next year, and my puppy fat has turned into a big, biting, non-house-trained bitch of a problem.

If a doctor had asked me (a little kid fed up with her chafing and boys only wanting her for her comedic skills), I would have offered to give him/her my last steamed chocolate pudding with white custard if they'd 'cure' me.

I started thinking about this conundrum when work asked me to read about the Fat Files, which is what I call the recommendations from those NICE (National Institute of Health and Clinical Excellence) boffins who've come up with loads of methods aimed at tackling record levels of obesity in the UK.

Under the proposals:

- The NHS will get the go-ahead to perform surgery on seriously obese children

- Local authorities will be told to provide more areas in which people can exercise safely and free of charge

- Schools must make it easier for children to lead active lifestyles as well as teaching them about healthy living

- Individuals will receive increasingly detailed information from doctors on how to remain healthy.

Nowhere does it say they'll give us free access to a gym, make personal trainers cheaper than chips, or make it law for ALL high street shops to stock clothes over a size 16. And then some.

I did the story and found a list of ideas that do make sense to me.

Having read up on it, it seems that I possibly could have been offered surgery back then, if these proposals had been on the cards some 20-odd years ago.

What if I had a child, though? What if he or she were big like me? Would I cart him/her off to the surgery and beg the doctor to 'heal' him (or her)? I wouldn't even consider it because I would hope that my child, chubby or not, was like I was way back then – big, but adored.

I know a girl who liked food but her enjoyment of it

was watered down by a mother who knew her daughter was bigger than average – in height and size but nowhere near gargantuan.

Her size 16 mother watched what her daughter ate, dressed her in clothes way too small (and old-fashioned, if you ask me), and told her she'd grow up to be ugly if she continued to eat chocolate or ate three pieces of toast for breakfast.

She also didn't really allow her to have friends over to play but was in no way tight-fisted or lacking in the generosity stakes when it came to material possessions.

And, whenever I saw her and went to the fridge to offer her something, you could see her pause before uttering, "I really shouldn't... Mam said I wasn't to have anything more today. She'd go mad if she knew."

And I'd tell her she was lovely – she was.

I'd tell her to have a little bit and remind her that what her mother didn't know didn't matter.

Maybe I was in the wrong but, having spent years secretly eating and then openly declaring my dissatisfaction with myself, I thought I'd be cheating every big child out of knowing one simple truth about themselves – they're lovely as they are, rubbing thighs'n'all.

Yes, of course it would be better if they were smaller, fitter, healthier. They're just not worthless if they're not.

That girl has since lost her 'puppy fat' – her mother, in her generosity, bought her an exercise bike instead of the laptop she wanted – and she looks wonderful.

In all honesty, she looks better than she did as a chubby child who was obviously uncomfortable in her skin, dressed in the wrong clothes and made to feel like a fat-faced freak if she put extra food in her mouth.

But making her feel bad then, as she was, was too

little too late.

In a sense, just like NICE's proposals, we are trying to make people slimmer when the barn door is closed and the fat horse is struggling to prance around the field.

So there you have it, then.

The basic truth is that on current trends, by 2010, an estimated 12 million adults – plus one – and one million children will be obese.

You'd think, then, it would be easier to shop for clothes. And that bigger kids wouldn't feel so rubbish about themselves. Perhaps, before surgery, we should dish out support on a giant plate along with the tools to feel good about themselves.

And people could be extra NICE by starting with this big baby first.

To ask women to become unnaturally thin is to ask them to relinquish their sexuality

Naomi Wolf

ONCE UPON A TIME, women wanted to look like Pamela Anderson.

Blonde, big haired and boobylicious.

She wasn't what I would call curvy, as she's still skinny to my mind. But at least she wasn't stick thin.

She had what the tabloid writers like to refer to as 'curves', which means a Jessica Rabbit type figure with a pinched waist.

But Pammy's whammies and her innie and outie bits are no longer aspirational body types; instead what passes for the body beautiful in America (and you just know it's going to filter down to us) is the skin and bone look which comes in at a dress size zero. Yep, zero for nothing up top. Or below.

Or in the middle. Anywhere really.

This mythical size zero is akin to a UK size 4. Have you ever been in a shop and seen a size 4? Realistically speaking, shouldn't it only be available in Mothercare?

And I'm not talking about the maternity gear here either.

The designer Michael Koors has said that women "are proud of starving down to a size 4. In Hollywood, nobody breathes what size they are unless it's a 2."

If you're as crap at maths like I am, you'll be delighted to know that there are sizes more inch squeezing than zero.

You can get double zero (look at *Desperate Housewives*'s Eva Longoria for that one), negative zero, XXS and even -2. MINUS 2! Isn't that a temperature?

I can't even contemplate the British equivalent to these microscopic sizes as my little head is starting to think of pink dresses that come tagged with 0-6 months.

I just don't understand why people would deliberately choose to be this small, this tiny and so inconsequential-looking.

These women don't just want to be slim, they want to be über dwti – that's the Welsh for crackers.

They want to be asked "Who did your breasts?" and answer that a Dr Dreamy did the reduction, not enlargement.

I've just read this article which states that, in LA, pipe-cleaner slenderness is the new black.

The shapely-does-it aesthetic which used to rule has now been sliced, diced and decarbed of its lustre

Instead of skin, bones rule. People like Nicole Richie (ugh), Victoria Beckham (why?), Keira Knightley (boobless wonder), the Olsen Twins (Mork calling madness, come in madness) and Kate Bosworth (is it me or does she look as if she's got the wrong-sized head on her shoulders?) define perfection.

These women, who were once 'human'-looking and certainly could pinch more than an inch (even if it was only a millimetre extra on their toenails) have obviously worked hard at looking so ridiculous.

Not for them a sensible diet, or walking up an extra flight of stairs a day to tone up and slim down A BIT.

No, reaching size zero 'perfection' (I am sighing here) involves some hard work.

You can't only look emaciated, you have to look toned as well – hey, I read that even Richie works hard at looking so ribtastic that she goes to the gym at least four times a week. Shit, who'd have the time?!

Me? I find it boring just walking up the stairs four times a week, let alone subjecting myself to a hard-core drill instructor who wants to see me literally sweat buckets and expose my hip bones and make my clavicles (no, not a musical instrument, I'm told) visible.

I don't even KNOW where they are on my body, for God's sake, but there are personal trainers in America who only deal with women who want the Nicole Richie look.

It's a sad day for 'normal'-sized or healthy-thinking women everywhere when people like Debra Messing, Gwen Stefani, Heidi Klum and Sharon Stone would rather hang out in New York as opposed to LA because they feel they're too fat for La La Land.

Too fat? I've seen chunkier KitKats.

As one anonymous stylist to the stars said, "Skinny isn't just a trend; it's the culture now."

Speaking as a body double for Bella Emberg and desperate to be made redundant, common sense tells even dissatisfied me that I'd rather stay at my fleshy best than play exalted hero at zero.

Even if that means being laughed at in the street in La La Land.

Anyway, I'd rather take a BIG bite of the BIG Apple any day. I've heard the portions are better there too.

"PAT? ANYONE SEEN PAT tonight?"… asked the slimming teacher.

"Yeah, I've seen her," said someone from the class.

"Where is she then? She didn't tell me she wasn't staying tonight."

Classmate, "Nah, she's had to go home."

Teach, "Oh, anything wrong?"

"No, she's just starving."

Picture it. Me and about 40 overweight women – some of them a dieting size eight, the freaks – falling about laughing at the irony of it all.

There were we, all sitting around waiting for the teacher to tell us if we'd been good girls (and one boy) all week, trying hard not to go Evil on the new Fat Club plan (six pounds in two weeks ladies… read it and weep for joy for me).

So we're there, all wanting to go home for something that's in our new food rainbow guide and eat 36 of them as they're guilt-free stuffing.

And one brave soul simply bolted because she was starving. Fabulous – you couldn't make it up.

Neither could you make up the next conversation.

Teach: "Diana, I see you put on two pounds this week."

D (name changed in honour of the Fat Protection

191

League): "I've been good though, really good, 100%."

Teach: "So why the weight gain, then?"

D: "I don't know. But I did have two take-away curries this week, four pints of lager, a packet of crisps after last week's class and a kebab after the pictures. Do you think that would do it?"

Teach, trying not to smile: "Umm... well... yes. What do you want to do for next week?"

D: "Lose 10 stone. Failing that, only have the one curry."

Slimming class is like society in miniature.

They're all there – fat, thin, successful, target weight girls, oldies, goodies, young women, obese, svelte, hopeful, defeatist, mothers and daughters and people, like me, who sit in the back hoping not to be made an example of when the time comes for Teach to read out what you've achieved that week.

It's the first class I've been to since that time in Ebbw Vale, years ago, where the ritual humiliation wasn't an exercise in helping out its members, but making them feel like pigs. Literally.

Slimming classes, as you know, have various ways of psychologically bolstering your confidence; conversely, because you're baring your eating soul as well as the numbers on the scales, they can embarrass you into activity.

But reverse psychology never worked on me, after I found out that my mother's warning, that my mouth would stay in an eating pose if I continued to stuff, was false. Well, partially.

Have I mentioned before that fabled class of mine where, if you put on weight, the teacher didn't say, "Oh, well, pick yourself up and shake yourself down... you're only human, so back on it next week in earnest," like my new guru does?

No, that one's unique method was to get you to stand up WEARING A PIG-SHAPED BADGE.

And when the teacher read out your weight gain, the rest of the class would oink at you. Yep, oink.

Talk about ritual humiliation – I don't know about you, but I can make a pig of myself without the help of sound effects or lapel accessories.

But this new class, this brave new world near home, feels different – or should that read that I feel different there?

I've only been going for two weeks and in that time I've moved from hope to disappointment to elation and back to hope.

The first week on the plan, I only lost one and a half pounds. To say I was gutted was an understatement.

But it was onwards and upwards as Hiya Love, the chief cook and chuckle maker of my life, continues to weigh out 42g of mozzarella and 200g of chips (but only if I'd had a relatively light calorific day), calculate how much pasta I could have if I was having a carby day or if I had enough grace left over to get me all clucky on a meaty one.

Crazy? You've got to be a little nuts to put yourself through this… or just desperate. I'm not convinced I'm either. But there's six pounds less of me mulling it over today.

Brain cells come and brain cells go, but fat cells live forever

Anonymous

HE WAS TRYING TO describe someone on work experience in the office.

I knew what he wanted to say – more to the point HE knew what he wanted to say – but he didn't have a clue how to get it out.

There were two women at work and one was tiny, almost child-like; the other was more – oh, here's a word for you – robust.

"So go on then, which one is the better of the two? I've got something to give out and I want a good job done," I asked him.

"The one is better than the other," he said, telling me what I already knew.

"And that one is?" I mused, knowing that what he was going to say was that either the smaller one was good, or the bigger girl was.

And he looked up at me, straight into my chest (I had the Top of the Pops camera angle advantage at this point) and mumbled something. Of course I heard what he said. So I asked again. Just for the sheer bloody hell of it.

"Which one? I need to know as I can't give it out if they're not up to it. Who's good?"

"It's the, er, um, well, um, bigger one."

All that fuss over one little word. The 'bigger' girl.

And she was bigger – about a size 16 I'd say, compared to the size 6 girl on the other desk.

All he was doing was stating a fact – but he must have thought that I was a member of Fat Feminists or something, the trouble he took about saying "bigger".

And then came the photo shoot. There's a game we play in work called Guess Whose Hands They Are.

Basically, in times of need, the snappers call on journalists to pose as models in pictures for the paper.

It's normally staged, done to highlight a story – you know the kind of thing.

Someone's written on, oh, I don't know, Welsh sausages, and they just get someone to bite into one.

Following?

The other day they wanted to shoot someone leafing through a calendar, so they found someone in the newsroom to go and pose for it in the darkroom.

For someone, read thin girl with manicured nails and something tight on.

Of course, nobody on the desk would admit to doing it, to being fattist (as if nobody big ever eats sausages. Hello?).

But to put this into some sort of context, the only time I've been asked to act as a hand/face/leg/clothes model was… oh, that's right, never. And I've worked there seven years.

When there was a fancy handbag story, did they pick me?

No – I guess that's because big women don't own fancy handbags.

Then there was the carrier bag shot, to stage a picture of where people shop – you know, Tesco vs Morrisons etc.

Was I asked? They looked up and down the newsroom, were turned down by three – three, count them – thinnies. And did they once think of asking me?

No, course not. Because big people don't go food shopping. Right? Well, in my case it is true as housemate Hiya Love does all the shopping, but you can see the point I'm trying to make. I'm not asked. Ever.

I'd love to think I'm overlooked because I'm far too important, too busy, or too damn wonderful. That's my mother's voice whispering in my ear there, the one which likes to think that everyone is born equal and we're all simply fabulous.

My head's doubting Thomas – otherwise known as the Fat Controller – is much, much louder, he rants and raves and says to me in his all-knowing way, "You're not asked because you've got fat hands. And that's ugly. If they wanted pork sausages, they've have gone to a butcher for some."

Granted my hands are like baby hams but when I once asked a friend if he thought my fingers looked like sausages, he looked at me and said in all seriousness, "Nah… I'd say more like éclairs, Han."

People just don't know they're doing it, do they?

They just don't realise they're making value judgements on face value. Literally.

My digits may not be good enough to be photographed, but you should see their grip – we're talking Olympic strength here when it comes to hanging on to a good old corned beef bap.

> **Strength is the capacity to break a chocolate bar into four pieces with your bare hands – and then eat just one of the pieces**
>
> **Judith Viorst**

AS OF LAST WEDNESDAY I've lost half a pound short of a stone in weight.

That's 13½lb in old money.

I got on the scales at my Fat Club class, Hiya Love watching me from the sidelines with one eye as the other pored over recipe books, nose sniffing out any gossip, when they told me I'd lost five pounds that week.

Five pounds! The week before it had been one and a half pounds, the week before that just one pound. To say I was gutted was like saying, oh I don't know, you'll get thin eating Chinese food with only one chopstick.

But last Wednesday, despite having some chips with a meal (chicken salad and a side of guilt) on the Tuesday, I lost just under half a stone.

It's taken me five weeks which, in Hannah time, translates as a lifetime.

Patience isn't one of my virtues – cleaning a plate is – but at least I'm giving this dieting thing a proper go this time.

On the whole, I'm good; when I'm bad, I quickly try to recover.

But do you know the hardest thing of all?

It's to not shout about my Olympian achievement and to avoid wearing a T-shirt emblazoned with my new weight – because nobody's noticed I look any different.

A stone for me is nothing I guess, in the grand scheme of things. It feels like I've lost it off the plaque on my teeth.

That was until my diet teacher handed me this great big lump of orange stuff and told me to feel it.

I did – horrible, smelly, huge, and definitely last season's colour.

Then she told me that what I had in my hands was two pounds of fat – and that I'd lost almost seven of them.

Count them again please – really slowly – seven of them.

The orange beast was launched on me and my unsuspecting but largely, er, large class mates for the first time a fortnight ago when, one by one, we were all bemoaning the fact that the most of us had only lost an average of two pounds.

"Two pounds? Is that all?" asked one disappointed woman on the scales.

"Bloody hell, the omelettes that I've been eating all week have been so light I've had to lay my knife across them and even then they struggled to stay on the plate. Which, incidentally, I borrowed from the dining room in my daughter's doll house."

When it came to my turn last week, and the sighs turned to collective applause for my relatively huge loss, I was bombarded with questions of how I did it, mingled with whispers of "lucky cow".

Stuck for words – as far as I could see, I didn't do anything that differently – I just lapped up the mass jealousy for a few minutes, knowing that next week my heart may again be on the floor as the scales reveal that week's reality.

The trick, when it comes to keeping a healthy and

realistic attitude to weight loss, is to take a stab at what the AAers do, take it one day at a time.

Because, if you remember to be patient while forgetting to be disappointed in yourself, a weekly two pounds loss over a year means you're waving bye-bye to more than 100lb of fat.

And that, in the cruel light of stones, tops more than seven of the nasty sods.

Just think of the stickers I'd get in my Fat Club fat book for being a good girl then.

It would be a veritable rainbow of achievements.

And we all know that somewhere over that half-hearted rainbow there may be a glimmer of light which will lead to a better, fitter, leaner, orange-free me.

> **No diet will remove all the fat from your body because the brain is entirely fat. Without a brain you might look good, but all you could do is run for public office**
>
> **Covert Bailey, US fitness expert**

I'M THINKING OF WRITING a book, the working title is How To Lose Your Lardy Arse And Regain Your Life.

It's going well so far – obviously, it's about me (no surprise there) and my battles with not only my bulge but the full-on fist fights with myself too.

It's going to make for uncomfortable reading, I think.

Chapter one starts, like Julie Andrews suggested, at the very beginning, a very good place to start. When you read, you begin with ABC – when you're a lumper, you begin with Please Feed Me. Now. Oh, and after. And all the minutes in between, thank you very much. Hey, time's got no meaning when it comes to calories.

It charts my early love affairs with beef dinners and Yorkshire Puddings the size of houses, and having a box – yes, a box – of salt'n'vinegar Chipsticks at the end of my bed to dip into as and when I felt like it.

And I wonder where my problems started.

From there, we move swiftly on to my life as it is now, 35 years on and counting (just like eating cakes, I'll poke my fingers into the filling in later chapters).

And where exactly am I now? Still dieting, still dissatisfied, still wishing I was more than I am with change left over.

I am, though, trying my best to be upbeat about it and

to think about the long-term possibilities of being healthier. My glass, though, is always half empty – positivity isn't high on my list of attributes. Negativity I have in abundance but I'm trying not to lapse into the old habits of being, well, me.

And that's someone who over-eats, over-indulges and over-estimates my ability to put things into perspective.

This week, for example, I was kicked in my not-insubstantial belly when I went for my weekly weigh-in at Lumpersville.

Last week, I'd lost five pounds, putting my total loss at half-a-pound off a stone. I stepped on the scales in the little hut, empty packets of crisps and biscuits littering tables and emblazoned with their calorific value (bad, bad, bad), tottering towards it like I was some glam gal with emeralds plugging the holes in my cheesy cellulite.

"Oh, you had such a glowing report in the class last week," said one jealous bird.

"See, we knew you could do it – but *how* did you do it, love?" went another.

And I'm answering them, smug in the realisation that I was just a few footsteps away from walking on those scales and seeing that half-a-pound – and more – slide away, and radiate success like a former chubby Readybrek kid.

My hair's looking fabulous – it has just the right amount of bounce – make-up is flawless and I'm thinking I must call up Bobby Ball to ask if I can borrow his red braces as my trousers are literally hanging off me.

All this is playing through my mind as I walk, no float, towards the scales thinking that I'll bottle this moment forever in How To Lose Your Lardy Arse And Regain Your Life, use it as a guide for all dieters who CAN succeed like me, whose life CAN change if they're good/wonderful/motivated/strong like me.

And I turn to the girls stood behind me, give them one last big, beautiful, aren't-my-cheekbones-sticking-out-more-now smile and step on. God, I can almost taste victory on the tip of my almost defunct tongue.

And I look down.

And I look up.

And I look down.

And, just like the *Countdown* clock, the ounces tick past me in slow motion.

And I hear this bell, this piercing noise in my heart, that tells me the weight is in. Just like my hips, the scales don't lie.

I put on one and a half pounds.

I put on one and a half pounds.

I put on one and a half pounds.

I PUT ON one and a half bastard pounds!!!

I stepped off feeling the jewels melt, my hair frizz, my make-up run and my heart deflate.

"Never mind, love – better luck next week," went the one woman.

"Remember, at the end of the day, there were people on the Titanic who turned down the sweet trolley," went the other. And at that moment I felt that it wouldn't have mattered if I'd been one of them, I'd still be back to square one.

I've been extra good this week, though, and the third chapter is coming on a treat. It's called I Keep Trying To Lose Weight But The Big Bugger Keeps Finding Me.

I've decided that perhaps I'm bulimic and just keep forgetting to purge

Paula Poundstone

I'VE LOST 17LB AND still nobody's noticed. I've even had my hair lopped off, thinking it would make my chin look thinner and my cheekbones resemble cheekbones instead of wishbones with fat on.

Nope. No takers so far.

Having picked my heart up off the floor after putting on one and a half pounds the week before last, in my last weigh-in I'd shrunk by a further three and a half pounds.

And that was even with a bar of Galaxy and a pastry-less quiche (like hard scrambled egg with bits in) the day before.

I've walked to the train station in the freezing cold; I even had chicken salad for tea while Hiya Love dished up his homemade lasagne for his train mates Ben and Jacky.

I didn't even make a fool of myself by asking to lick their fingers after they had finished.

God, that was hard. Not only do I tuck into a satsuma while the smell of pieces of granary toast the size of doorstops wafts around the newsroom every morning, I had to say no to his Italian work of art, worthy not only of tasting but on-your-knees adoration.

I'm a wonky, difficult to please foodie but I say, hand on heart, that Hiya Love is a wonderful cook.

I also put my 17lb loss largely down to him.

Because he's the one who panders to me; he's the

chief chef and shopper in our house.

He's the saint who cooked me lasagne made out of swede pieces instead of pasta sheets when I was on the Atkins.

He sieved off fat when I put my hopes and jeans into Rosemary Conley's plan.

He went to Tesco late at night for two dozen fresh eggs when I was on the yolk-only plan.

He didn't begrudge a large part of our shopping money being spent on Special K and Bran Flakes when I went through a stage of eating cereal for breakfast, dinner and tea.

What can I say? He's a real man. Because – sigh – he's the one who weighs out my chips. What wouldn't YOU give for a man who not only cooked them for you, scraped out the filling of a Chicken Kiev as you're on a parsley-free day, but who also weighed your chips?

"And cooked them from scratch, love," he's forever reminding me. "None of that frozen rubbish."

With him, everything's always from scratch. Just like his stories that I've heard a hundred times before.

He tells me he can see I'm losing it (no irony there).

He is my calorific counter, the one who tries to keep me on the straight and (hopefully, please, one day) narrow when I feel down about this thing called my Fat Life.

OK, so he may be the messiest bugger in the world – why use a spoon when you can use 12? – and the one time he cooked steak at my mother's house my father said he had to put the high-powered wash on the kitchen tiles.

But so what?

Apart from my father, Hiya Love is the only man who's ever weighed out my chips.

And I simply can't count the ways to say thank you, Love.

All of the things I really like to do are either immoral, illegal or fattening

Alexander Woollcott

I WANT A CHEESEBURGER. With bacon on.

You know, one of those really fat ones that look like a mountain.

I'm fed up, fractious, and I want to eat. Badly.

I want to eat for Wales, eat for a tiny English village, eat 'cos it's Wednesday, eat for ever, eat because I don't want to forget how to chew. Come on, it could happen…

I'm not sure what it'll achieve, apart from putting on some of the 19lb I've now lost (I'm still a size 24 too – how does that work?).

And feeling like hell.

And getting annoyed with myself.

All over a bloody cheeseburger.

Healthy-minded people, as I like to call non-emotional eaters, wouldn't go all out for grub when life's getting them down and turning their innards inside out.

They'd simply suck in their feelings, sort them out, maybe take an extended toilet break to think about stuff, have a cup of coffee and move on.

I just go to the loo to avoid mirrors and unhinge my over-shoulder-boulder-holder out of my nooks and crannies.

Other people know that issues affecting them are, well, smaller than them in the long run.

Me, big bugger that I am, can't imagine anything being larger than me. Except a house that is a triple-decker with room for a caravanette which sleeps a family of seven out the back.

Today, for instance, I've tried to be a walking, talking, example of restrained humanity.

I smiled at work at this bloke I kind of know, who I like to call Cement Clive to myself.

He came over to me, all teeth and chin and cock-eye (like one's in Brynmawr and the other's in Tonypandy, as he talks to me).

And I listened patiently as he droned on about himself – my pet hate, apart from skinny portions, fish, calorie counting, summer, dieting, sweaty thighs and weighing scales.

But no, I thought, be nice – put your best face on, show that smile girl, be good to those around you and goodness will surely follow you all the days of your life (or some such nonsense I recall from chapel).

Then I won't dwell in the house of fat faces for ever, no doubt.

Then came a call from Significant (thin) Other, who intimated that my ego was the size of my ample arse.

And, as anyone who knows me will tell you, that is kind of wonderful.

We were discussing photographs of me for a special project, pictures for the cover of this book.

He said that a particular picture which he wanted to use was lovely; trust me when I say I looked like the love child of Hell and Back in it, with more chins than a Chinese telephone directory visible for all to see and throw darts at.

I informed him politely, for he was doing me a giant favour, that I wasn't keen on this particular image of my fleshy phizog and would it be possible – pretty, pretty please – to use a different one.

"But people like you when you smile, they'll relate to it," is how he put it.

"I agree. It's just that I don't like that picture of me and I've lost quite a bit of weight since then," I countered.

"I can't work with someone with as big an ego as yours!" was his retort.

"I don't have a big ego, just a big arse," was my trying-to-make-light-of-it response to such weighty matters as which picture of me to show to the world.

And from then on, because I'd upset him because he'd upset me about the whole ego thing, and because I'd upset myself, the day started to go horribly, horribly wrong – or rather, my mood did.

Cement Clive, obviously deluded into thinking he was on to a winner and I'd suddenly turned into sugar-coated Hannah, came back up to try his luck again with the second part of his story about the day he went home on the train.

And it was late.

And he missed his favourite homes show on the telly.

It was about Redruth.

And he had a shed which had a red roof.

And that made him laugh.

Which it didn't me, of course.

So not being a total bitch, only a bit of one, I did the secret eye signal to a sympathetic pal over the other side of the room, the one which screams RESCUE ME NOW!

And she called me, pretending to be someone with a story, throwing me a life-line which safeguarded him from getting verbally trounced and me from being thrown out of the building for my language.

He left, I sighed, we hung up.

And I went into her office to effusively thank her for

the save, my body feeling a little perplexed after my 27th day of jacket potato and baked beans for lunch. (No butter, heavy on the crispy and wind.)

Only to be greeted by a sight which strikes fear into the clogged arteries of insecure foodies everywhere – for lunch she was eating a cheeseburger.

With bacon on.

You know, one of those really fat ones that looks like a mountain.

I managed to keep a civil tongue in my head, but it took all my super sized strength not to stick it out and lap at this carby altar for solace, even for a few moments.

But the ego, I think, has landed. And it's parked in a space marked Volatile.

The leading cause of death among fashion models is falling through street grates

Dave Barry

THE CONTRACT I SIGNED with Beauty was obviously written in invisible ink.

My concept of 'self' – don't worry, I'm not going to get all, ahem, heavy – is a higgledy-piggledy commodity, one that can often be found in the bargain bucket of my worth.

This, and my concept of how attractive I am, is inexorably tied to how I look. This, then, affects how I feel.

Topsy-upside-downy thinking? Yep, with a cherry on top.

The other day I went on the scales in Boots. I always do this just before I'm due to have the Fat Club weigh-in on a Monday because I need to know, quietly to myself, if I'm going to feel like shit or like Superwoman on the night.

It's always a few pounds 'out' compared to the digital wonder I greet at the start of each week at Fat School, but I figure that any loss is a loss. Right?

So I stepped on, a feat in itself because I have to go in, hope nobody is in there drinking methadone while staring at me, take off more layers than should be allowed in a public place and try to stop myself from either doing a dance (if I've lost) or breaking down (if I've put on) and, guess what?

I was the lightest I've been in a zillion years.

210

I felt elated, overjoyed, and started to wonder where I could get coasters printed at such short notice with my face and weight on.

There was nobody to share my good news with, so I trotted back to the office feeling lighter, brighter and bigger in the self-confidence stakes.

I settled into my seat convinced that my arse was no longer hanging over the sides like congealed beef dripping, when an email binged in from FC.

It announced that I was last week's top dieter, and that they'd keep a sticker for me (bless) and my name would go on the Wall of Fame and stay there for four weeks.

And I'd only lost two pounds! Which meant my chip-weighing Sisters must have all gone home gutted and cried into their fridges as they'd only managed to shed a sliver.

Because I'd left early, said Teach, she'd had to give my prize to the woman who came second in class.

What was it, anyway? I knew I wouldn't be congratulated with a box of chocolates like a normal person celebrating good news or a personal victory.

Hey, maybe it was a voucher? A recipe book? Magazine subscription? You know, anything I couldn't EAT?

Nope, a bowl of bloody fruit. FRUIT!

I hate fruit. Too much hassle getting to the goods if you ask me.

I don't mind strawberries (if the tops are cut off and they're already washed for me), red apples (as long as they're polished like the really shiny ones in *Snow White*), or bananas (hard as nails and almost green, please). But there it stops.

This was the first time I'd ever been given a bowl of fruit as a mark of success. I mean, talk about a sick joke.

Anyway, I told Teach I didn't mind, no bother (thinking I'd rather suck on a Fisherman's Friend – and I'm not talking about the sweet there), and the weight loss and accolade was enough in itself, I gushed.

So there I was, coming over as a mild-mannered and frankly better-looking Naomi Campbell, when it happened.

The Slump.

From feeling fine, I suddenly sank down into the shit of feeling like the pits.

There's rarely any warning, no notice period, just an all-pervading black dog called Inadequacy that snaps at my heels just at the point where I think it's started to appear well-trained.

Five days later, I still haven't managed to claw my way out and it's weigh-in day tomorrow.

In the thick of it all, I took Hiya Love and Mr Hannah out for a meal.

In 'The Slump' already, there was nothing I could do with my hair/face/make-up/clothes/frankly crappy attitude to make myself feel batter – oops, better (sorry, I had Yorkshire Puddings on my mind there).

When in 'The Slump', I become someone else entirely.

I'm quiet. I'm reflective. I'm sad. I'm fat. I'm fat. I'm ugly. I'm fat. I'm unlovable. I'm ugly. I'm fat. Can I get cream with that?

I also forget to remember about my 19lb weight loss, about Boots, about my sticker, about anything positive.

And I eat. Stuff for Wales, and the guilt is palpable.

Instead of thinking, bugger it, I'm out for a meal and I have been good for months now so I'll just have a little treat and not worry about it because – and here's the clincher I can't quite grasp in this life-long battle of

212

trying to feel better – tomorrow is another day, I order garlic mushrooms to start, steak and chips for mains, and jam suet pudding with custard for the sheer bloody hell of it.

Hiya Love and Mr Han know what's going on, but they don't dare say anything because I'm sensitive – certainly to criticism and definitely to anyone, however well-intentioned they are, who mentions me and food in the same breath.

So the Ugly-ometer is rising, beauty barometer's getting low, and according to my internal sources, there's only one place to go.

No, not to join the Weather Girls as the third, fatter member, but eat more.

The next day it's cousin Owyn's first birthday party at my mother's and, almost magnetically and certainly blindly, I'm led to the kitchen where I open every cupboard looking for boiled ham like some demented sniffer dog.

Mam Jones finds me skulking and although she's the only one in the world who can comment on my Lardy Arseness, whose look of disbelief can crush me into a thousand little insignificant pieces (just like the way I love salt'n'vinegar crisps in a sandwich… see, I'm off at a tangent again), she knows I'm in 'The Slump'.

So she BUTTERS me four mini rolls which she fills up with boiled ham and vinegar.

I eat these while standing up and telling her, mouth full of absolute wonder, that I was (Top Secret) stones on the scales in Boots.

"That's nice love. Do you want another," she looks up at me and asks, hoping I'm going to say no so that I can get back on track.

"Yeah, ta Mam. Just two more as I've got to weigh-in

213

on Monday. Got any crisps? Anyway, you should have seen my face in (chew) Boots! I was (chew) over the moon. I didn't (swallow) have anything to eat when I (chew) got home in the night then and (chew) did I tell you I was slimmer of the universe in (chew) class? I could have had fruit (guzzle) as a prize. Last night we (chew) went out – can I have a tomato please? – but I only had a (liar!) chicken salad as I'm being really good and it was a nice place (chew), you'd like it. Can I (lick lips) have a piece of cake? Just a little one (I'll sneak another later when I pretend to clear up). I can't remember the last time I had a piece of (chew) cake (last night, remember Han?)."

And I ate subconsciously, ate with lies littering my conversation, like some recovering alcoholic who thinks a spotlight will beam down on them if they even so much as look as a can of Shandy Bass in the Spar.

Instead of simply enjoying what was on offer, the dissatisfied dieter in me couldn't put a forkful of food in her mouth without feeling fear.

"To eat is a necessity," said La Rochefoucauld.

Yet to eat intelligently is an art.

But to be honest, I was never much cop at drawing.

I am a dab hand at feeling less than I am, however.

And I'm not talking in terms of inches, unfortunately.

> **I developed a nutty attitude where I'd think, if some guy really loves me he doesn't care if I'm fat. I'd come up with all these stupid reasons why it would be OK to be fat**
>
> **Kirstie Alley**

I STUMBLED UPON THIS programme yesterday about a girl – size 12 if I'm being generous – who did this experiment to become a size zero.

She lost something like 18lb and dropped two dress sizes in a couple of weeks. To be honest, I'm jealous – I've lost half a pound short of a stone and a half and I'm still a size 24. Where's the science in that?

I mean, I know there's no justice in the world but this is just plain cruel.

The other day, feeling inspired because my hair was probably sticking up in the right direction, I thought I'd go into Evans and – gulp – try on some size 22 trousers.

And I did, and they kind of fitted, and I left with two pairs of black wide-legged beauties and some skinny jeans. Not the type of skinny that make girls' legs look like pipe-cleaners gone wrong or men bandy as if they're on the wrong side of rickets, but skinny as in fitted.

And I'm there, in the changing rooms, thinking that I've seriously got it going on because I didn't have to contort or place six mirrors around my face to see all of my chins.

I suspect they have 'thin' mirrors in the changing rooms, like they've been borrowed from a bazaar based in a land far, far away called Dreamersville.

Anyway, with a fantasy mirror this way, that way, behind me, to my left, to my right, encircling my obviously shrinking fabulousness in a Trinny and Susannah type showdown, I also notice that said chins are disappearing.

Where I don't quite know, but I'd hazard a guess they're in a waiting room some place, just hanging on for the opportunity to reattach themselves if I fall off the wagon and into a world made up of Wagonwheels.

Anyway, chinless wonder that I am becoming, I slip on the skinny jeans. And they fit! I could almost cry for joy. Instead I go out to show Mr Han, who is sitting on a settee with all the other Fat Admirers by the lingerie section.

"What do you think?" I ask eagerly, already putting the answer in his head.

He was supposed to say, "You are a vision of beauty, skinny jeans were made for you; your belly's disappeared, the shape of your legs is goddess-like, you look a million dollars and then some. Come quick, let me lick your face you beautiful, desirable beast. By the way, where have your chins gone?"

Instead he did the worst thing he could do, well a few of the worst things, actually.

He didn't fall about in admiration, he didn't leap up and propose marriage or at least offer to pay for the jeans, and – look away now if you're of a nervous disposition – HE LIFTED UP MY TOP TO SEE HOW THEY HUNG ON MY BELLY.

Got the ENORMITY of that? If I'd had the energy, I would have demanded he section me there and then under the Crimes Against Fashion Act.

"Don't do that!" I screamed. "It's not as if I'm going

to wear the bloody things with a bolero top and bold gold jewellery, am I?"

And then the realisation of what I'd done, of how I'd try to dupe myself into thinking I had it going on, suddenly dawned on me.

I'd been in a daze, obviously hypnotized by the magic contained in the mirrors.

For the purposes of my sanity and in a subtle bid to convince myself I was now a full-fledged 22-er, I'd cunningly pulled down my top over my belly to hide the small planet that it has become. Unfortunately there was nothing I could do about the camel hooves.

So I suddenly developed a stoop, but I hoped nobody would notice, as I attempted to do that shoulder-shrugging stance, like I'm too cool for school and always walk with my head to the side (hey, I needed more length immediately, and hoped I'd contort myself into gaining 3ft of extra material to cover the damage).

I then made sure I was able to get back to my changing room WITHOUT having to turn around so he wouldn't see my arse, packed up as it was like a cannonball in stretch denim.

And he said, with an unwittingly clear swipe at my sanity, "Don't worry, you'll fit into them soon."

"They fit now! Look! Can't you see? You must be bloody blind then, because I'm in a size 22 AND I can bend down in them," hoping at that moment nobody dropped something because, frankly, I'd have split more than my heart open on the floor had I dared to bend (and I don't bend for anyone, let me tell you) to pick it up.

Anyway, I got the trousers and took one last look at my (lack of) chins before heading into Monsoon.

There I continued my charade of thinking I was finally what I've always wanted to be – and that's a high class,

High Street shopper.

I slipped into the changing room with two tops, both a size 22. Here the delusions took on a different form.

So what if the bottom set of buttons didn't do up on the one? You don't need to do them up, was my convincing excuse to myself – the fitted nature of the blouse made that wonderful dip in my back more pronounced and my waist look tiny (well, you know, relatively speaking).

And who cares if the sash on the waist of the other one wasn't supposed to sit under my boobs, but nestle gracefully on my waist? I'm certain that the Jane Austen look is in – there are enough re-runs of Pride and Prejudice on the telly, anyhow.

This time, Mr Han ooh'd and aaah'd in all the right places, even offering to buy me the two pieces of hope in 100% cotton.

I didn't succumb though, didn't do what I've done all my life and get them, hang them up somewhere to look at, as if they'd give me inspiration to lose enough weight to be able to fit into them one day.

Nothing, not even a 40% press discount card for Evans, to get what the hell I want in whatever fantasy size I fancy, has that kind of power over me any more.

So I left them there, and instead went home with my skinny jeans and two pairs of identical black trousers.

But do you know the curious thing? They're hanging up, for me to look at, giving me inspiration to lose yet more weight. Still.

Self-delusion is pulling in your stomach when you step on the scales

Paul Sweeney

"OH, THAT LOOKS HEALTHY," she said, as I munched on a yoghurt.

"Don't know," I answered in between mouthfuls (I had to be quick as I had three tubs open and I didn't want any of them to go off, did I?).

"I was told in Fat Club they are golden food. So I have, on average, about 10,765 a day now. Give or take."

"I guess it's the calcium in them, the Omega this and thats which are good for you then," my slim friend offered.

"Umm… well… haven't got a clue what's in 'em. I don't ask questions after hearing the words 'you can eat as many of these as you like'."

She came back with, "I'm trying to be good too. I've started to alternate a packet of cheesy biscuits with carrot sticks."

At this point, never having tasted a carrot but certainly having played that game of stuffing a load of cheesy biscuits into my mouth to see if I could talk with a dry gob, I wondered, for the umpteenth time, why really slim, lovely looking girls, with bodies to die for and hair made for a Timotei advert, are so strict with themselves.

"Why are you being good?" I ask, confusion written all over my face, now in a Lasting Satisfaction (please!) strawberry yoghurt type-face.

"Have you seen your figure? If I had a body like yours and wasn't prone to putting on weight, I'd be stuffing all the time."

"Because... er... well... I suppose it's because I'm trying to be healthy."

"Healthy? No bugger can see your innards!" was my twisted logical argument back in her beautiful face.

Funny, isn't it, how differently people see the weight thing.

Whenever people ask me why I want to lose weight and why I'm on yet another diet, I always say it's because I want to live a healthier lifestyle.

My body, I tell them, is a temple (albeit one already semi-condemned with a few cracks in the roof).

I don't give people the real reasons which can basically be reduced, just like a good bolognese sauce, to a few home truths, tossed in a not-so-light Hannah style dressing.

And that's because I feel ugly, I hate not being able to buy stuff on the High Street, and I want to see my feet.

This is my unholy trinity, otherwise known as the Three Little Pigs of Me.

When you say you're on a diet, that you want to lose weight, for whatever reason, I'm sure that most women think I'm doing it to reach an absurd goal weight, some space age size.

Here's an admission – for those who missed it the first time: I DON'T WANT TO BE A SIZE 12. I don't want to be the kind of slim where I'd be capable of touching my toes – as far as I'm concerned, if God had wanted me to do that, She would have put them on my knees.

I don't want to think of carrots as a treat, either. Carrot cake, however, would make me think twice

Not afraid of heights – afraid of widths

Anonymous

WHO DID YOU WANT to be, Cagney or Lacey?

I, greedy as ever, wanted to be both; I wanted Mary-Beth Lacey's cheek bones but hair like Christine Cagney, follicles you could yank at in the toilets and come out looking fabulous.

Luckily, I was into *Cagney and Lacey* during the 80s, when I was too old to re-enact scenes with friends, but still young enough to dream of a hard-nosed life like theirs.

I loved the way the two women interacted and the general buzz of the show, although I wasn't really aware of its pervasive melodramatic overtones at the time.

Ha! Look at me, like some half-arsed anthropologist. Don't worry, I think I read that sentence somewhere before.

It was just good cops going after baddies, but this time in tight jeans, a fluffy jumper and good shoes.

I only got to appreciate its depth years later.

Questions of appearance – dress, body weight, hair styles – were constantly under consideration and negotiation by the producers and stars themselves.

Story material, particularly when focused on issues of vital concern to women – rape, incest, abortion, breast cancer – often proved controversial and led to continuing battles with the network and many column inches in the papers.

Personally, I shouldn't have minded being cast as

either Christine or Mary-Beth, had I still been young enough for play-acting.

They were both feisty, both ballsy, both hard in that soft kind of way self-confident women are.

Looking back, when it came to picking playground roles, I think I would have been stuck with Mary-Beth because, let's face it, she was the less glamorous of the two.

She had flats, Christine walked over criminals in heels; Mary-Beth's husband Harvey had a moustache the girth of which members of the Village People would have been proud; she wore a dirty mac to work while Christine pranced around in either a fur coat or leather jacket with the collar up.

I wasn't what you would call an unattractive child, but I certainly wasn't a small one.

I towered over my friends, and would try to make light of my lack of lightness by showing off my strength in other ways, acting the toughie with a kind heart when all I really wanted to do was be one of the girls that the boys fancied rather than laughed with – or, worse still, laughed at.

I was always in with the 'in' crowd though, a gaggle whose constituent members were all clever, cheeky, chopsy, sensible, daring, sporty, musical. We were the Ebbw Vale equivalent of the Bash Street Kids, only with cleaner knees.

We used to go down Ian's house to watch videos and I can see myself now, idly wasting time talking to the adults while everyone else clambered into chairs in his living room.

I didn't rush for the best one, because I was scared to death I'd sit on one and someone else would want to share it with me. And I didn't at the time know how to amputate my arse in order to facilitate this.

It happened just the once, the seat sharing incident, and it caused quite a stir among my friends.

There was Lee W and I sharing the best seat in the house, the one facing the telly.

We cwtched up the best we could, me not exactly sitting properly but trying to look like I was comfortable watching a two-hour film at a wonky angle.

I was caught out, though, when Lee wanted to get up to go to the toilet, only he was jammed in. With me. And my arse.

I tried to wiggle out of the wonk and into the straight and narrow, but all I succeeded in doing was working up a sweat.

We eventually worked out that if we both moved at the same time, in the same direction, with the joint aim of detangling his hip from my mine, we could get up.

So on the count of 1, 2, 3, heave-oh no, we managed to stand up together – only to realise that the chair had come with us too.

Oh how we laughed; and oh how I cried with the shame when I got home.

I was about ten at the time, with a ten-year-old's sensibilities but a fully grown woman's bits.

Reconciling the two was heartbreaking for me.

It was my grandfather who told me I was unconditionally beautiful. He didn't say things like I was lovely ANYWAY or DESPITE being big.

I, with my mother, was the most precious thing in his life. I was brilliant, funny, and my bare arse sticking out of the bed clothes in the night wasn't a sight for really, really sore eyes.

I can hear him whispering to my nan now, thinking that I was asleep, about my 'big, beautiful full moon' of a bottom, the sight of which brought such joy to his life.

When my other friends and I played Charlie's Angels, fat-faced and clumpy-shoed me was never allowed to be Jill Munroe or Kelly Garrett.

No, it was always pudding-haired, clever-clogged, sensible Sabrina for me.

And I'd go home, depressed with legs chafing as usual because I refused to wear jeans bought from an adult shop, complaining to my grancha about the injustice in my little world.

He'd squeeze my cheeks – oi, the ones on my face, cheeky buggers! – give me a big kiss that seemed to contain all the love and goodness in the world, and say Sabrina was his favourite anyway.

Today, aged 35, I still think of myself as that kid who never got the plum part, often talking myself down instead of up.

Because of what I do – I tend to think it's because of this, and not because of who I am – I could be moving in some of the fanciest circles in Wales on any night of the week.

Circles, which I'm sure the Jills, Christines and Kellys of my past would give anything to be part of.

Instead I'm thwarted by my own sense of insecurity, thinking that even now I'm not quite good enough to belong.

Maybe that's because I think the chief excitement in a woman's life is spotting women who are fatter, uglier and worse-dressed than she is.

I, for one, refuse to be anybody's Sabrina.

Because as Patrick Swayze said in my fantasy version of *Dirty Dancing*, "Nobody puts Hannah in the corner."

(Unless we had a chair each, that is.)

> # The French fries taste like smoked plastic, they just taste like this completely fabricated thing, this long, yellow thing
>
> **Morgan Spurlock**

HOW'S THIS FOR THE most boring conversation in the world.

Hiya Love: "How did you do, love?"

Fatso Jones: "I only lost half a pound."

Hiya Love: "Better on than off, love – I mean, better off than on."

Fatso Jones: "Hmmm... gutted though."

Hiya Love: "But it's going in the right direction. And you did have two Yorkshire Puddings at your mother's on Sunday, and two scoops of swede mash. And last night you had a bread roll."

Fatso Jones: "Don't forget the one piece of toast I gobbled in one gulp."

Hiya Love: "See! That could explain it, love."

Fatso Jones: "What, that one piece of toast, two Yorkshire Puddings and a bread roll would have left me feeling like a useless waste of space? Most people eat that in one go. Shit, I would normally have had that while waiting for my salad to, er, saladify."

Hiya Love: "Han, you may be geographically in the Valleys, but psychologically speaking you're in denial."

Fatso Jones: "Bugger off. What's for my tea anyway?"

Hiya Love: "A sense of humour on Ryvita?"

Fatso Jones: "Bugger off. It's just that I hate talking

about this all the time; I hate weigh days, I hate sounding like a stuck bloody record, I hate this ruling my life. God, I used to be interesting."

Hiya Love: "No you weren't. But you were BIGGER. Get it through your fat – sorry – thick skull. You've lost 21lb for God's sake."

Fatso Jones: "No I haven't, I read the book wrong. It's 19½lb. Check it for me, will you? Just in case. You can go in and get a sticker for me then."

(Hiya Love turns on the light in the car and with his CSE Grade 76 in maths counts up the pounds.)

Hiya Love: "No, they're wrong, you have lost 21lb! What colour sticker do you want? I'll go in and tell them now."

Fatso Jones: "What about the one and a half pounds I put on that one week? You have to count that. 'Cos I think without that, it would be 21lb – with it, it's 19½. See? That woman with the glass eye was right – it's one and a half pounds to the stone and a half."

Hiya Love: "Oh… right… well, it's still loads, isn't it? Look on the bright side, love."

Fatso Jones: "No thanks, I chafe in the sun."

Hiya Love: "You miserable cow."

Fatso Jones: "Don't you mean miserable FAT cow?"

Hiya Love: "Just don't have toast this week and we'll go back to weighing your pasta."

Fatso Jones: "Weighing my pasta. Has my life come to that? Am I really resigned to thinking that a balanced diet is a doughnut in each hand?"

Hiya Love: "You're just a nutritional over-achiever and if you want to make yourself really depressed, you should ask to be weighed in grams next time. Your trouble is you want it all now. And you know you've never stuck to anything. You've always had it too easy, love."

(F)at which point I was about to launch into my theory that in fact I am very much hard done by (sob) when I turned and caught sight of a girl from Fat Club – a really important one too, as she sells the biscuits – ordering sausage in batter and a bag of chips from the Chinese.

Having spotted me, the smile on her face slowly dripped away like the stringy cheese on a pizza. I could see her hold her stomach in, and stand more upright at the counter as if telling me that cheating is only cheating if she actually did it on a Wednesday.

Maybe the chips weren't hers, I thought to myself, giving Biscuit Monitor the benefit of the doubt; perhaps she was buying them for a relative and was going to go home, like me, and have a bowl of rice flavoured with protein-heavy hope.

So I'm sat there, the taunting aromas of chip fat and chicken chow mein wafting towards the car, when she did it – the Shoulder Shrug.

In case you don't know what that is, it's the upwards motion of said shoulders, a simple purse of the lips, and tilt of the head to the left that all guilty eaters do when they've been caught out with their hands in the cookie jar.

It's like a 'whaddya gonna do?' ambivalence, a sign that yes, you've been naughty, but it's the kind of bad that's going to taste so very good.

Almost three months into the diet and 19lb lighter, I haven't succumbed to The Shrug. Yet.

I've been close; I've been so dangerously near to the upwards motion, I could almost taste – oh, there's a lovely word – its flavour between two pieces of bread and a packet of salt'n'vinegar crisps. I may even have had one shoulder up, until I finally came to my senses and realised that I get enough exercise just pushing my luck on the scales every week.

Out of professional courtesy for a fellow foodie, I almost yelled out to her that I really know my chips, was an expert in the field, and could help her judge their flavour on a scale of Fabulous to Heavenly.

But at that moment, realising that yet another milestone was only one and a half pounds away, however I massaged the numbers, I thankfully remembered where I was, what I was hoping to achieve and that a bag of chips with all the crispy bits at the bottom wouldn't make me feel better in the long run.

She walked out, held her bag of treats up high for me to see, and The Shrug followed the tick and tock of my inner calorie counter.

Fatso Jones: "19lb lost. It's not bad is it really?"

Hiya Love: "Not bad? It's bloody amazing love! Now, are you on a meat or veg day today? Because I thought, for a special treat, you could have a couple of chips tonight... "

The slimming industry sells the obvious to the indolent

Camilla Cavendish

I CAN'T MOVE, WHICH is surprising since I've been on a stealth mission for the last hour and I handled that just fine.

I can safely say I out-manoeuvred anyone who knows me or would recognise me.

Because in my hands – stop, it's worse than that – in my hands AS I WAS WALKING, was a Burger King meal.

Then a cheese and onion pasty from Greggs.

I'm sorry. Honest. I'm really sorry.

I'm saying that to the precious 19½lb of me that I've lost and to everyone who's said to me over the last few weeks how good I'm being – crazy, crazy fools – and how proud they are of me.

So why did I do it?

Why did I walk in to the burger joint then walk quickly back out again £3.99 lighter with a bag of food in a paper bag, like some fat wino with no self-control?

Why then, obviously not sated but on a (deep filled) roll, did I think about a Mexican chicken baguette (with cheese, of course) from one of the arcades?

I only thought better of it because it was busy and I was running (now there's a laugh) late.

How come I settled for Greggs instead, a place which always makes me feel nervous – not because I could run (sorry, amble) riot in there, but because I never know my place in the queue?

I may be pushy, but when it comes to grub even I don't shove.

I don't understand it.

I was fed up when I woke up and I'm still on the dark side of dandy, to tell you the truth.

It's been rumbling, unlike my stomach, as that seems to be full all the time lately, for a few days.

I'm fed up and fractious, so maybe I was just having a weak moment.

I'm only human, right? I mean, isn't it entirely reasonable for me, the feminine painters and decorators about to move in for a week, the disappointment of only losing half a pound this week, pressures of work piling up, to seek a little pleasure?

The trouble is, I'm not reasonable with myself.

As I beat myself up about being a bread bimbo, I notice that Mads behind me is tucking into an apple, cabbage, walnut and fennel salad, which is my idea of hell.

But it is guilt-free eating in its finest, glowing, I'm beautiful and you're-a-porker-Han, form.

Sam, on my left, has just bought a bag of oranges from the market, a punnet of strawberries, and did so ON THE WAY BACK TO THE OFFICE FROM THE GYM.

Karen's had a Shapers meal deal from Boots, Paul's on sushi, Gareth's nibbling carrots, and Cath's picking at something green.

As for me, I've still got pasty crumbs in my teeth as well as on my blouse, sticking to me like yellow dandruff. It seems I don't use the head on my shoulders to think straight about my dietary life.

This week, as you're reading this, I'll be in London so I won't be weighing in.

The dilemma of what to do there has already started – and I'm not talking about which show to go to.

Should I 'diet' when I'm on holiday? Or should I be halo-inducing good, knowing that, if I am, the week after, as I approach the scales, I'll have a veritable spring in my step, honestly believing that I'm edging closer to another personal half-milestone?

I can't just 'be' in the moment, take things as they come, because I'm fearful that if I take the foot off the accelerator of my motivation, the slimming engine that drives me will conk out for good.

And this is all because of a pasty. And a Burger King meal deal. Stuffed when walking.

On days like these, when I feel disappointed in myself, isolated and invalidated, my life's menu sadly doesn't consist of the two healthy choices – that of just taking it or leaving it.

> **Getting my lifelong weight struggle under control has come from a process of treating myself as well as I treat others in every way**
>
> **Oprah Winfrey**

TODAY'S EXCLUSIVE STORY: DIET secrets of the stars!

Thought that would get your attention. Everybody, it seems – bar me as it happens – wants to know what so-and-so does to stay slim and look good.

There's so much written about what the beautiful ones eat, don't eat, what exercise plan they're on, what trainer they go to, what detox plans they advocate.

So there's got to be some magic secret, right? Some potion or advice they get when they become members of that club called Chafe Free?

Come on, do you really think that if you eat eight mini meals you'll look like Jennifer Lopez?

Or that, if you become vegan, you will you eventually morph into Alicia Silverstone? Will sipping green tea make you a Claudia Schiffer-alike? Will you get a face like a 10lb trout like Melanie Griffith by only drinking smoothies, morning noon and night?

Will John Travolta leave Kelly Preston for you because, like her, you eat shed loads of oatmeal and bagels?

And will you ever be in the 'Zone' like Jennifer Aniston? And I don't mean sneaking into the Parent/Toddler one in Asda's carpark.

Like shoes, celebrities come in all shapes and sizes. You've only got to look at the variations in the diets they follow to know that there's only one truth when it comes to trying to understand how they do 'it' and keep 'it' off – there ain't one.

As Buffy star Sarah Michelle Gellar put it, "Look, it's crazy for people to try to be as thin as we are. We have personal trainers and personal chefs. It's our job to look this way."

And it's our job to measure our self-worth against them.

Wake up and smell the burning a tight pair of knickers makes on your arse – these are human beings we're talking about here, not supersonic women who know it all.

The difference between them and us lily-livered mortals is that they work with people who have the ability to make a magic trick look like it was sent in a box from heaven.

Most of them, it has to be said, have good genetics. They're fab-looking, smart, and know how to play the business they're in.

And in case you don't know what that is, it's the one where they get paid to look good, even if on the inside they're crumbling.

Look at Oprah Winfrey. She's one of the most successful women in the world, certainly one of the richest, but she's struggled with her weight for years.

Like me – yes, I am going to mention her name and mine in the same sentence, which is the closest I think I'll ever get to sitting down and asking her how the bloody hell she's done it – her issues stemmed from a bloody big hole in her psyche.

"I know it appears I have everything," she once told an interviewer from *Ebony* magazine, while glancing around her $20 million, 88,000-square-foot film and TV complex just west of downtown Chicago.

"And people think because you're on TV you have the world by a string. But I have struggled with my own self-value for many, many years. And I am just now coming to terms with it.

"As I peeled away the layers of my life, I realized that all my craziness, all my pain and difficulties, stemmed from me not valuing myself. And what I now know is that every single bit of pain I have experienced in my life was a result of me worrying about what another person was going to think of me."

She even blamed being fat on the scurrilous rumours which flooded America that her boyfriend Steadman was actually gay.

"I believe in my heart that, had I not been an overweight woman, that rumour would never have occurred," she said. "If I were lean and pretty, nobody would ever say that. What people were really saying is why would a straight, good-looking guy be with her?"

When she lost 60lb, she told *Ebony* that her real joy was realising that she was "finally ready to let the weight go. Not the pounds. But the weight of my life.

"My weight was always my apology to the world," says Oprah, who works out twice a day and had a personal chef and trainer to help her lose the weight properly.

"It was my way of saying, 'OK, I'm rich, I've got a good-looking boyfriend, and I've got this great life, but, see, I've got this big weight problem so you can still love me.' "

Like many of us with a weight problem – how I detest that phrase – her real issue wasn't with the fat but sorting out why she never felt good enough to feel lovable – for who and what she was, inches'n'all.

As she told Laura B Randolf, "The other day I was jogging down the road and this woman said to me, 'You better quit losing so much weight because you're going to make the rest of us feel bad.'"

"What she really meant was, 'Listen, if you start looking better than I do, I'm not going to like you any more.' Well, I'm finally ready to own my own power, to say, 'All right, this is who I am. If you like it, you like it. And if you don't, you don't.' So watch out. I'm gonna fly."

We, though, can only look on in wonder, betting extra on the Lottery, hoping our numbers will come up so we can bag ourselves a chef and personal trainer just like Oprah.

Then, we say to ourselves, we'll get this thing sorted out once and for all; then we'll have the tools to help ourselves.

I've done it – I've given myself intellectual incentives, thinking I'd be onto a winner IF ONLY I had a personal trainer and my local Tesco had Quorn.

I've thought about how I'd refocus, regroup, re-evaluate my position (normally lying down on the settee, granted) if my circumstances were different, if I had Angelina Jolie's lips to make sucking cabbage soup through a straw sexier, if only Catherine Zeta-Jones would call me and share her Hollywood secrets about looking and feeling good.

But as you know, there isn't anything to divulge.

Because we're all different, all wanting, all needing to feel more than we are, even the people we call 'stars'.

It's just that some are maybe better at moving in the right direction.

As Oprah said herself, "Do the one thing you think you cannot do. Fail at it. Try again. Do better the second time. The only people who never tumble are those who never mount the high wire. This is your moment. Own it."

Celebrity food for thought...

Halle Berry

"I eat healthily and don't eat a lot of junk food or fried foods. I've found that balance is the main key. I notice a big difference in my attitude when I'm exercising. I'm more confident and much happier."

Jennifer Lopez

"There are a number of weird diets out there but I don't follow them. I eat almost everything, only in moderation. I totally believe in having a healthy well-balanced diet. On the fitness front, I'm not a fanatic. I work out when I feel things getting jiggly."

Gaby Logan

"I wouldn't say I'm obsessed but I am aware of my diet. I know what's good for me and what isn't. If I'm going to have a blow-out I'd rather do it on something I really like. I don't feel guilty because if you do you don't enjoy your treats."

Melinda Messenger

"I've devised my own five-minute crunch workout and I do it naked to really motivate myself! Seeing the bits I'm not happy about wobbling spurs me on to do something about it."

Emma Bunton

"Keeping fit is key for me. It's all about tweaking

your lifestyle. For example, I was doing sit-ups in front of the football on TV the other day. I got so excited I had to do something!"

Gwyneth Paltrow

"I gained 35lb when I was pregnant but my mother told me, 'You can't diet when you're breast feeding'. For the first few months I didn't lose any weight but when I started doing pilates and yoga, it came off."

Jerry Hall

"Everything in moderation. I drink lots of Evian and sleep a lot, at least 10 hours a night. I eat three well-balanced meals a day. Skipping meals just means the body saves up fat. I don't snack and I avoid alcohol as it ruins a woman's appearance."

Claire Sweeney

"When I was 17, at the Italia Conti stage school in London, dancing every day, all day, I never really thought about my weight. In fact, I was too thin. I was eight-and-a-half-stone and I'm 5ft 8ins. Now I've got to watch what I eat. I organise my food before – usually low fat snacks and a ready-meal to pop in the microwave at lunchtime. In my tea break I try to munch on fruit or reduced-fat crisps."

Sharon Stone

"I bake all the time, but I don't like to eat the cookies when they're done. I just like the dough."

Beyoncé Knowles

"I lived on water, cayenne pepper and maple syrup for 14 days. It was tough; everyone was eating and I was dying. After that I ate waffles, fried chicken, cheeseburgers, French fries, everything I could find. That was the best time of my life. I've gained twelve pounds."

Eva Longoria
"I go to the gym at least four times a week to stay in shape. Before the show I might have gone once a week. Now there is pressure because people recognise you wherever you go."

> **The voice of intelligence... is drowned out by the roar of fear. It is ignored by the voice of desire. It is contradicted by the voice of shame. It is biased by hate and extinguished by anger. Most of all it is silenced by ignorance**
>
> **Dr Karl Menninger**

I CAN'T WAIT TO scrub myself free of the day. Had I the pathology, I'd take a scouring pad to my face and just rub until I could safely say I was starting again.

Clean plate. New head. For certain.

I've reached an uncomfortable impasse with myself, one that I recognise from my past and, it seems, my present too.

The future – my dieting fate – looks grim today. And, if I'm honest, I've been struggling to keep pace with the pace I should be going at to get where I want to go – keeping up? – for a while now.

So I scrub; I take off my make-up, which doesn't seem to be doing me any favours these days, I mess up my hair that now looks like an orange version of ridiculous, and I take off my work clothes. In an odd twist of logic, the only sort of clobber that gives me any real respite is sportswear.

How funny is that? Some bright spark must have been out jogging one day during their lunch hour and idled past a load of suety arses spilling out of their jeans, and thought to themselves, "Oh... If only I knew someone who could sew 12 of my tracksuits together and make them into something one of this lot would wear. Wonder if they'd buy it?"

Only you don't get Juicy in sour sized couture.

So I'm in my comfies, those stretchy comforters that wash like rags and just happen to look like them on me, wondering how to silence my unrest.

My mind just won't keep still; it's a silly little tool that gets me into all sorts of trouble with myself. Don't get the impression that I stand idly by and let this happen, though. I fight it, I rally against it, but still the balance is tipped in the direction of defeat.

And it's all about balance, isn't it? It's all about finding what works for me and sticking to it, re-learning the rules of my life, addressing my wonky attitude to food and myself, or accepting that if I really, truly deeply can't change me, then I need to find ways to change the way I think about myself.

I thought, you see, I was doing OK. So, all right, I haven't reached that stone-and-a-half loss yet as I cocked up the numbers and, sue me, I had that pasty and Burger King meal the other day. But, by and large, I've been good and felt fine, positive, thinking I'm on my way to a better-looking and -feeling life.

To what, then, do I attribute the blame of this internal rebellion? Dysfunctional thinking, perhaps. But is that too deep?

Isn't my ability to stay focused and interested in myself (now there's a new thing) just that? I have no staying power and I have no patience with myself. And I just want to say "Fuck you then, Jones" with chips. No, with Chicken Kiev. Pizza would be good too. And garlic bread. Baked beans, beef-burgers and fried eggs with potato waffles. Corned beef rolls. A packet of crisps.

Fruit'n'Nut. Family-sized. Chewing gum. Sweet milky tea made with full-fat milk. Afternoon tea with scones and little sandwiches. Cereal. Rhubarb crumble and custard. Chicken salad. Noodles. Fried rice. Boiled rice. A liquidized Mars. Toast. Anything, as long as I didn't have to dissect WHY I was having it first.

Good or bad, I don't care what it is tonight, as I'm feeling pissed off, and I just don't want to have to factor in a diet. I want to eat and feel normal. I just want to indulge in a little sugar-coated Nice biscuit without having to kiss guilt's big fat arse afterwards.

The start of my cholesterol-fuelled thinking started the other day when I got an invitation to go on a photoshoot in London.

It was for a really big newspaper, and I'd get to plug my book they said. All I would have to do was try a new diet drink – something coffee-flavoured, flown in from Norway.

I'd drink it three times a day for a month and it would, apparently, speed up my weight loss.

They needed a 'before' snap and for me to reveal to the world, how much I weighed and what my measurements were.

Frankly, I would rather give out my sort code and account number.

The best is yet to come, though – I'D HAVE TO BE PHOTOGRAPHED IN A PAIR OF SHORTS AND A T-SHIRT!

So I wrote back saying I couldn't do it, that revealing my vital statistics was one thing – they're big, but my hips and boobs are ten inches bigger than my waist giving me some semblance of a good shape (well, at least from the front or back…) – but posing in shorts was too much for me to contemplate. Way too much.

I'm writing the email, and in my head I'm imagining the picture and the boys in the office laughing at me; millions of women going "poor dab… she must be desperate for the money – you'd never get me in shorts"; my mother wondering yet again why the hell I put myself in a position where I'm famous for being big.

The journalist came back quickly, saying she'd had a word with the picture editor and the pictures would be "tasteful, after all this is the Fancy News and not the Daily Take Off Your Bra" and I could wear cycling shorts. Would that make a difference?

Honestly? It made things worse because I started to hate the fact that, yet again, people were making allowances for me.

Luckily, I have souls around me who see more clearly than I do, even with a new prescription. In their wisdom they pointed out that I couldn't buy this kind of publicity for my book, the £200 fee would come in handy, and I'd get to be 'glammed up' for my 'after' shot in the paper.

I thought this all sounded good for a while, until I started to stare Mystic Meg-like into my future. There I found myself standing before a rail of clothes some cock-eyed stylist had picked out for me, one filled with drop waists, geometric patterns, leggings and stone-washed denim WITH a matching cropped jacket.

What if this happened, I asked myself. What if I got there and I had no choice in what I wore? Would I, my self-belief shrinking by the second as I faced powerful types in fitted trouser suits, feel strong enough to say, "Actually, you lot can bugger off – it's tunics or nothing. And if you think I'm wearing leopard print you can think again, sunshine."

In the end, a matter of crediting me as a journalist for the Western Mail made the decision for me – they were willing to cite me as an author, but not someone who works with words on another publication.

I'm never going to look like Daisy Duke; I'm never going to be happy in shorts or relinquishing my power over what I wear.

So I may have stood in my bedroom and rolled up my trouser legs just to see what my exposed calves would look like, and I may well have shaved the buggers for the first time in about ten years.

But still, when it came down to it and push came to shoving me against the wall of my better judgement, I couldn't go out and 'celebrate' my 'curves', which is what they tried to convince me I was doing.

I don't have curves, see – I have runny fried eggs with hats on for boobs, a belly that is like a giant inflatable doughnut and thighs that are one rub away from igniting.

For me, it's not about looking like a supermodel; it's about feeling good about who I am naturally. And naturally, I don't come wearing shorts and a T-shirt.

I come damaged for sure, but I also come knowing that I'm nobody's stooge.

Except, perhaps, my own.

> # After all, people die, computers crash. All we can do is breathe and reboot
>
> **Carrie,** *Sex And The City*

I'M FACING THE BIGGEST dilemma going. Should I go back to Fat Club tomorrow after two weeks off the diet knowing that I'm bound to have put on weight; or should I try to do this on my own? I mean, I've got all the books now. Right?

Mr Han, looking at me sympathetically before reminding me of his "you've been on holiday" logic, says I should go back, grit my teeth and just accept that I've been, well, just human over the past fortnight. A – gulp – weight gain is inevitable.

I'm not so sure if I can follow that thought process though.

Hiya Love, for example, brought bread home today – brown bread, "just in case".

"Just in case of what?" I goaded him.

"Well… you know… just in case", he said, mouth contorting into a shameful grimace which translated as I Know What You're Like But I Don't Want To Be Cruel So Brown Bread Is Better Than White In The Land of Denial.

"Don't worry, I won't eat it," I said, dipping some into his sauce for chicken chasseur (he was positioned in front of the serving hatch as Mr Han was out there waiting for his dinner, in full view of my dipping action which I've perfected to supersonic speed.)

"I'm only having a piece (three in fact… I don't count

crusts, see) today because I'll be back on it tomorrow. Might as well enjoy myself today as I've not had a good fortnight, what with being on holiday and all. One (three, remember) won't hurt me."

But hurt me it has. It's unsettled me. It's made me feel like I'm back to square one. The bread of my personal heaven has turned into a hellishly slippery slope and I feel I'm sliding back into my old ways, as I demolish more slices.

This, in turn, brings me back to the Fat Club conundrum. I don't get anything from it any more – but the fact that I have to go there every Monday and go through the ritual of payment, line up, look down, leave with either a spring in my step or dragging my heart on the floor, to phone everyone in my mobile to break the bad/tell the good news, did get me into some kind of routine.

I've done it for three months now, which, when you look at it reasonably, isn't that long really.

I've been good, really bloody good, I've felt positive – well, as positive as negativity allows.

But how easily I have fallen at the altar of carbs.

It all started, like all memorable journeys, on the train to London. But let's go back a step or two.

When I was little, it was a running joke of my parents that I would eat my egg sandwiches by the time we got to Pontlottyn when we took the train from Rhymney to Cardiff to go shopping. (Ponty was the next stop.)

Move forward 30-odd years, and there I am, all excited because I'm on holiday AND THERE'S A BUFFET CAR!

Now I could, of course, have opted for just a cup of coffee or, if I was really pushing the dietary boat out, a latte made with full-fat milk.

I could have said, when Mr Han offered to go up and get me something, no thanks, I'll wait until our evening meal.

But what did I do? I took a deep breath as I knew there'd be no stopping in this sentence and went with a straight up, "I'll have a sandwich thanks but only if it's nice bread but if they have baguettes up there and you don't know which one I'd prefer bring back the two and you can have what I don't want and a packet of crisps would be nice, I don't mind if they're salt'n'vinegar or cheese and onion but I'm not fussed on those oven baked ones as they're too crunchy and they don't break up that nicely when you crush them in the packet but if that's all they've got they'll do but don't bother with chocolate as I don't want to be piggish and a drink would be nice – full fat one if they have it – and check out those breakfast rolls as Justin recommends them but I don't like sausages and only get it if the bacon is really crunchy as contrary to popular belief fat girls don't like fat on meat as least I don't, and you know, for the sandwiches right, I don't like pork, beef, anything with mayonnaise on, mustard, pickle, brown sauce, did I say mustard? Just don't be stingy, OK? Remember, I haven't had bread for three months!"

So I sat there, dreaming of the perfect sandwich/crisps/drink combo, the Pontlottyn of my mind racing back to the days when I didn't have to THINK about food or attaching such significance to the simple act of asking for a sarnie, when he came back with IT, a dream with a plastic flap.

A ham sandwich (just the one) and packet of crisps.

That was on the Monday. By the Tuesday I'd had a pizza, a salad, a muffin and a boiled egg, two semi-skimmed lattes, one bar of chocolate (I didn't suck, but let the warm milk do its magic dance in my mouth, convincing myself I was actually eating it slower and, therefore, digesting it at a healthier rate) and walked about 20 bloody miles (Mr Han does this... he deliberately gets lost so I'll have to walk an age in order to coax my food off, but doesn't tell me that's what happening – I'm too thick to realise it until my feet start bleeding).

Anyway, a week later and I'm starting to feel that this could be the end of my beginning because I've been bad; Mr Han says I've just been slightly naughty. But there's no normal human behaviour for us foodies, no definable middle ground called Graze.

So what if I've put a few pounds on? It's not the end of the world, is it?

No, realistically speaking, it's just a small mound in the mountain of my dietary life. Putting a few pounds on is child's play; getting it off is positively pornographic.

Dieting's dirty, it's hard, it's mean, it's degrading, it's vile.

And I guess that's why I'm going to swallow my last week of normality and try to get back into the swing of things.

For well over the 69th time in my life.

I'd kill myself if I was as fat as Marilyn Monroe

Elizabeth Hurley

IF THERE'S SOMEONE WHO really, really rubs me up the wrong way it's Liz Hurley.

I'm not sure what it is about her that winds me up so much, but she does.

It's not because she's rich, beautiful, successful and now smug married.

I think it may, though, be based on the reasons why I don't mind her pal Elton John's music but can't stand to look at him – she's unadulterated, ostentatious without the excess fat. Elton, on the other hand, just screams over-indulgence.

I remember reading a magazine article on Hurley (not so) Burly. During the interview she was asked to comment (read 'gush') about her boyfriend Arun Nayar.

I can't begin to tell you how many times she corrected the poor dab holding the dictaphone about how to say Arun.

And no, in case you're wondering, it's not pronounced like the jumper.

Itchily, she said it was like "A'rooooon". That's five O's if you're calorie-counting and forgot how real numbers work.

Christ, if I had to go about correcting people who dropped the 'H' with considerable aplomb every time they turned me into an Anna, I'd have to give up work to start a job in the pernickety factory.

It was the way she did it that got my goat, like it was a mortal sin NOT to know how to say his name the Indian way.

I mean, do we Welsh get pissed off if nobody can pronounce cwtch? When Dai becomes 'die' on GMTV *Today*?

Well, OK, we may do… but I'm sure you can see where I'm coming from here.

Anyway, aside from her marbles in the mouth accuracy, then comes The Look, the most annoying thing of all about her luxuriance.

Exhibit A: how ugly was that safety pinned Versace dress she's famous for almost wearing?

Exhibit B: how annoyed were you when you heard her, at the end of every edition of *Project Catwalk* on Sky One, tell a designer they were only knitting with one needle and had to go because "fashion has no muh'cee"?

Exhibit C: didn't you flinch when you saw her turn up at a friend's wedding wearing a scarlet dress split to the groin over a diamond-encrusted leopard-print G-string?

How upstaged would YOU feel if you were the bride?

Exhibit D: on a scale of one to ten, do you think it's mad for a 41-year-old mother to admit to eating just one full meal a day and snacking on six raisins, then saying watercress soup is a staple of her diet?

Which leaves me wondering where all the other sensible women in the world have gone. Were they invited to her 876 weddings to A'rooooon?

I've got to wonder, because women, 5,000 of them in fact, have said that her body is their favourite.

Yes, out of all the bodies in all the chip shops in all the world, they're most jealous of hers – they want one just like it. Only this baby can't be bought over the counter at Monsoon.

The sometime model, actor, film producer and swimwear designer is, I think, about a size Fabulous, one of those lucky buggers who manages to be stick thin but curvy at the same time, just like Kate Winslet and Katherine Jenkins who both look lovely.

But – and here's the deal she signed with fame – IT'S HER JOB TO LOOK THAT GOOD.

She's made a career out of having boobs that touch the sky, for god's sake, and a belly you couldn't balance a magic marker under when standing up. (Write in for tips if you're off to a hen do.)

A'roooon's other has admitted as much herself in the past.

The editor of *New Woman* magazine, where the survey was published, said, "Ordinary women can comfort themselves with the fact it is a 24-hour-a-day job, requires iron determination and probably very little food.

"For most of us, a body like Elizabeth Hurley's would require a lifetime of sacrifice."

Hey, giving up fried egg sandwiches is a big enough sacrifice for this woman – being career beautiful and not being able to fill up my car in Tescos sans bra, just in case the paps take a snap of my babs, would make my life a living hell.

I have to admit, though, that I DO think she has a wonderful body, I DO envy those curves, and I WOULD like to get a lifetime of Estée Lauder cosmetics as I hear they do a nice line in cellulite-busting cream.

But I just can't get it into my thick skull why people hanker after the largely unattainable, as epitomised by Ms Hurley.

To make matters worse, voters seem to have gone from the sublime to the ridiculous by voting Victoria

Beckham in at second place.

From 'curves' to the poster child for the pouting anorexic, it seems UK women don't really know what they want in their dream body shapes.

Posh paws may look OK from the front, but she's never going to melt a Malteser between her thighs, is she?

Former Hear'Say star Myleene Klass was third, who again is someone I'd call a shapely thinnie, but spirit level model Kate Moss also made the top five.

But there's good news for all those over a size 16 – Fern Britton made the list.

Whoopee! Pass me a pork pie now. Let's all celebrate the lovely Ms B coming in at a measly 93rd.

New Woman's editor Helen Johnston revelled in this piece of news with an effusive, "The variety of women voted onto the Body Idol list is extraordinary in its breadth – from the tiniest size zero to far more voluptuous celebrities who women admire and secretly envy for being comfortable in their own skin. It's also great to see such a high percentage of women over 40, showing that a sexy shape doesn't have to disappear with age."

Yeah, whatever. I'm 35 now and the only thing that's disappearing about me is the hope of ever being a size 18.

Another survey in the same magazine states that 97% of women think that anyone over a size 12 is fat.

If that's the standard, 99% of all the people I know, love and respect are porkers.

And I must look like an unwise Buddha in obviously crap-at-magic big knickers.

> # Sometimes you have to be a bitch
> # to get things done
>
> **Madonna**

Before Jacky

I'M NOT GOING, I'VE decided.

I don't really know what's come over me, but I don't think it's brightly coloured.

I've decided – deep breaths now – not to go back to Fat Club.

Frankly, my nerves won't stand it. I know I've put on weight. It's not that my clothes feel tighter or that my cheeks are hitting my eyebrows on the rare occasion that I smile these days.

Some things a girl just knows. I don't want to go on the scales in front of everyone and have the weigher do that thing where they just point at your fat book with the tip of a pen under the You Weigh This Now Sucker category, as if speaking the words "you useless fat lump of lard – what have you been doing this week, then?"

I'm feeling decidedly anti-social too, a whisker away from hermetic really.

I think it may have something to do with the clocks going forward and my mind swaying into reverse faced with these extra hours of daylight, hours spent when being SEEN.

Oh, I can just smell the cotton-tinged fear of wearing sleeveless smock tops as I write this.

I've also been told off by someone for not enjoying

252

last week's Burger King bacon double cheese burger washed down with a cheese and onion pasty, or, at least, for eating it without feeling guilty about loving every single bloody delicious fabulous fantastic tantalizing mouthful and then going, "Nice… right, it's back on the diet now."

Common sense doesn't compute, in case nobody's noticed.

Bread and dripping may just about make sense to me in this state of mind, but I'm a hedonist with a fat free conscience on this occasion.

Fat Club has served its purpose though. It's kick-started the low battery of my self-esteem and helped me lose one-and-a-half glorious stone.

It just doesn't hold my interest any more. The trouble is, though, where there isn't self-interest there isn't much hope of sticking to this dieting lark, for me at least.

Some people are natural born stunners/killers/dreamers/optimists – whereas I was not so much born under a wandering star but came out shooting blanks at the moon.

Sure, being funny about being fat and funny can be amusing in the right light; put my big life in the spotlight, though, and it looks like a giant pustule of full-fat cream that could explode over my brain at any moment.

Why, then, can't I simply accept that attendance at Fat Club has come to its natural end for me?

Because I'm worried not going will see me eating for company and not for pleasure, mixing up my carbs with a side of proteins like some ham-fisted disco DJ who can't get a gig because her name's not on the VIP list. Know what I mean?

On the other hand, I have simply had enough. So I say to myself, Han, you're a grown up, you've come this far,

YOU CAN DO IT GIRL! Give me an 'H', H!! Give me an 'A', A!! Give me... you get the picture, right. (Oh, gimme gimme gimme a man after midnight who'll drive me anywhere for a strawberry milk-shake please! It would take the shadows on my arteries away for a bit a least.)

I can hear the voice of Mam Jones, however, reminding me that I never succeed because I don't stick at anything.

"You gave up Brownies 'cos you didn't like the uniform, you played netball for Gwent but couldn't be arsed to go further because you felt you were too tall... what about swimming? Oh yes, you didn't like wearing a swimming costume because you felt too fat. If you'd gone swimming, you might have lost weight!

"Then there was the clarinet/saxophone/bass guitar, roller-skating, a hundred diet classes – your father could have papered the bungalow with the wall charts he made for the egg diet – photography, cookery and dance." Oh my.

After Jacky

I'm going back to Fat Club on Monday.

Jacky told me to, and I don't dare argue with the force of nature that is Mrs T (with as much bold gold jewellery as her more muscular namesake).

I get to the train station and she's there, in all her uncomplicated glory, laughing and joking with Hiya Love, bruising the air with her language not just turning it blue, standing chewing gum like a naughty schoolgirl with adult sized hula hoops in her ears.

Jacky is one of those people the term 'heart of gold'

was invented for. She's brash, bolshy, chopsy, mouthy, crass, common as muck, and simply mind-blowingly tender.

And under no circumstances would I mess with her, unless armed with a crate of cold lager and a £50 voucher for Top Shop to blind her concentration with.

She's like a good bra – close to your heart and full of support.

So I'm there, face like a ripped dap, a smacked arse – I can't measure misery – telling her I've suddenly become strong-willed and am not going to Fat Club any more because I'm capable – honest – of losing weight on my own, when she does that 'yeah right, who do you think you're fucking kidding?' face before launching into 101 reasons why I shouldn't pack it in.

Folded up water-tight like the casket that contains my Fat Club book, her argument was a simple one really, which basically came down to the fact that if I've failed on my own in the past, I'm bound to fail again.

She also reminded me that despite being able to sing in five languages, I obviously didn't learn to bellow out "No" in any of them.

At least, she said, I have a focus (only there were many more 'F's in her sentences) every Monday, otherwise known as weighing-in day.

Then came the crunch punch to my conscience – she'd go with me.

She, in all her size 12, 5ft 6ins, garrulous glory, would go home late to her kids and husband every Monday, just to give me support.

There's nothing in it for her of course, just the pleasure of my company and frankly I've known more entertaining amoeba on present form.

She's just doing it to help me, to comfort me, to

champion my record-breaking attempt at being a successful member of the Weight Loss Gang.

So I'm partially back on track, partly out of fear, and a smidgen out of respect, for someone whose concern for me is bigger than my lethargy.

And the last time I looked, it was covering the view of my feet.

A diet is not a piece of cake

Anonymous

EASTER, A RUBBISH TIME for an agnostic on a diet like me.

I didn't have any eggs, baring three fried ones over the weekend and four on a salad.

Not much fun, but at least they were without sin on my current plan.

Since then, though, things have gone from OK to sliding the wrong way as I crashed head first into a cheating daze.

From being slimmer of the week again – another two and a half pounds gone which means that I've lost over one and a half stone now – I've reached that all too familiar juncture where I simply forget to be good.

Not that I'm as bad as I was – I just lose context.

I was talking to someone about this the other day, about having 'time off' at Easter and other special occasions.

If I was thinking straight, I would know that it's fine to stray into the direction of beef-burger rolls done on the barbecue (three); a baked potato (one, medium sized) with sweetcorn (a tin) as an accompaniment to chicken (bad, bad, bad, mixing carbs and protein); one bar of chocolate (small, and it was Easter and I was feeling deprived – no, not depraved as I left that for a very, VERY Good Friday); lasagne and chips (I was out for a family meal, goddammit); and a large mocha in the coffee shop (skimmed milk and half the normal amount of chocolate).

257

All over a week, mind.

But because I'm the kind of girl who isn't fat, just too short for her weight at 5ft 8ins, I just slipped into the 'I'm a failure!' mind-set before the stray onions on my baps had time to solidify.

And I'm not talking the ones in the rolls there.

Now any regular person would think that my little indiscretions are nothing out of the ordinary, that to slip is fine as it's just a sign of being human.

I think I must be a Handriod then because when I slide I go so far into the sonic land of Insanity that I have to hitch a ride on two buses, a train and a spaceship just to get back on the right side of me again.

I've reached the conclusion that it's not slipping that's my problem, it's just not thinking it through properly and then, in the words of Mam Jones, picking myself up and shaking myself down and not dwelling on stuff too much.

It's my inability to go "oh well then, you ate so much your cereal dish came with its own lifeguard but onwards and upwards now, Hannah Marie Jones."

My two steps forward *always* equate to 8987 back.

I may be getting closer to wearing Levis 501s, but those measly beef-burgers on the barbecue have me thinking that I'm actually closer to Levis 50001s.

It's at times like these that I seem to conveniently forget that every day for the past fortnight I've walked to the train station (15 minutes and getting faster all the time); and when I don't walk, I'll do the same amount of exercise on the bike in front of *America's Next Top Model* (watching skinny women pout it out is cheaper than therapy and you don't need to book an appointment).

So how come I can't put just basic living and its sticky (toffee pudding… sorry, I was dreaming there) business into a workable perspective?

Some say the glass is half empty, others claim the same one is half full.

I don't drink, but I'd have to admit that I would say, in this present state of mind, are you going to swallow that love? If not, pass that baby over here.

But things are looking up. I had an email from the head of Fat Club today, literally the biggest loser in all the right ways, who reminded me that I'm just six pounds away from losing 10% of my body weight.

Sounds a lot, doesn't it?

Yet I can't help thinking that when you have 7686% of your unindexed mass to shed, 10% sounds like I've got rid of two zits and squeezed a couple of blackheads.

The thing about spots, though, is that they always come back.

But I'm trying my best to remain a champion squeezer, by staying away from picking at the beef-burger pile at barbecues.

> **When we lose 20lb… we may be losing the best 20lb we have! We may be losing the pounds that contain our genius, our humanity, our love and honesty**
>
> **Woody Allen**

UPBEAT TODAY. DON'T KNOW why.

It's sunny out, that state of weathered affairs which usually has me running for a dark hut in the hills.

At this moment, though, it's lifting my mood – if not my belly – and I feel like I'm the living embodiment of a Katrina and the Waves song.

You know, like I'm walking on sunshine instead of doing my best to avoid it. I don't have a reasonable explanation for it, however.

I'm also feeling positive, and not suicidal about the two pounds I put on last week.

Yeah, and gasp all you want at the news, but I know what I did wrong – I had food, stupid, stupid me – and just slid into that usual rut of feeling uninterested in myself.

So I had more food. See? Simple formula when you think about it.

Feeling utterly rubbish, I almost didn't to back to Fat Club last Monday because I didn't want to face the reality.

I don't want to taste (ooh, such a wonderful, fabulous word there) shame.

But go I did, only to stand third in line in a queue where girls walked up to the scales one at a time and punched the air with joy as pounds fell and their confidence grew.

Then came my time at the top of the big-bottomed buggers, my reluctant turn on the scales of doom where the news of the gain came in digitally.

"Sorry," I said to the weigher under my breath. "Not had a good week. I chewed all I fancied but forgot to spit it back out again."

"It's all right," came her kindly retort, and I swear I could see an empathetic tear in her eye.

"We've all had bad weeks."

And with that throwaway sentence, I regrouped.

Despite the two pounds, I'm still a stone and a half lighter than I was three months ago.

I just forget to put this in context sometimes.

A recent shindig helped me out a bit on this score.

I saw two friends the other day who couldn't get over the difference in me, which lifted my spirits as nobody else mentions it.

Mam Jones says it's because people in work see me every day – it doesn't explain why pal Justin didn't comment on it when we recently belly bumped into each other, despite standing like I was glued to a spirit level. And we hadn't seen each other in ages.

The Steves – try to keep up now, they're two blokes called Steve who live with each other – came over the other night, the first time I'd seen them since Christmas.

And they said I looked like a different person.

"Oh, and where have your tits come from? Darling, you are seriously sexy tonight!" went the younger one.

Older Steve, differentiated from his lover by the fact he wasn't wearing fake tan with fitted go-slower stripes running (literally) down the side of one arm, added, "Yes, you can see the difference. It's falling off you! You

261

must be a size 16 now."

At that I nearly choked on my lasagne/chips/bread roll/onion rings/garlic bread/cake/diet red pop combo I had for Hiya Love's birthday meal (but you know I don't like to waste food).

"Size 16? I'm still exactly the same size clothes as I was the last time I saw you!" I said in between mouthfuls.

"Rubbish," they bellowed in unison.

The one who's been Tango'd going, "As we've always said, it's not the size of the ship, it's the motion of the ocean that's important and you, darling, are moving like a demon on the dance floor."

In actual fact I was going up to the bar when I realised my top was caught in my knickers, so I was trying to get it out by acting like a contortionist with gout, but that's another story.

Neither did I feel guilty for having a 'proper' meal when we were out – I'd been really good all week, I'd done a bit of exercise and I'm so fattastic and fat-free living at the moment that I'm looking like a corned beef salad with red hair.

So I felt justified in a tiny blow-out, rather than standing out by asking if I could have a salad off the lunch menu at 8pm.

Maybe I'm on the evolution diet.

Frankly, today I couldn't care less.

I'm just enjoying it for what it is at the moment, because I know that internal good vibes are only six packets of crisps away.

I DON'T THINK I'LL be going to Topshop to see Kate Moss's new clothes range.

Jacky, on the train yesterday morning, dressed all in white like some high end ice-cream seller, suggested she take me "to have a nose" now she's found out the lot is coming to Wales.

She was no doubt thinking that a trip to Topshop would be a great way to celebrate the fact that I've now lost 10% of my body weight, a hefty two stone (four pounds off last week, girls).

What she doesn't get, however, is that I'm still a size 24 (I was also a size 24 two stones ago) and I don't think Kate Moss's thigh-scarring Daisy Duke shorts would do my left ankle justice.

Because that's what the biggest size would fit. My left ankle.

But try telling Jacky that; try telling her, even in the international language of sign where I stick my two fingers up to her when sound reasoning fails, that even if I COULD fit into a pair of La Moss's shorts and team them up with some fluffy ankle boots, you'd have to knock me out to get me into the shop in the first place.

I just don't get it when women over a certain age want to dress like their teenage daughters.

Leave that to the Americans I say.

Anyway, this is how the conversation played out

between me and the formidable Mrs T.

Me: "You look nice."

Her: "Yeah, I know."

Me: "Your wedges are good."

Her: "Yeah, I know. You wanna get a pair. A tenner these babies cost me. You should see the pink ones I got on the weekend. They're the wrong size, mind. But they only cost £3. Can't ask for more than that, can you?"

Me (scratching my head): "No, don't suppose so. Wish I could wear nice high shoes."

Her: "You minger, you want to start wearing them then. Like my trousers?"

Me: "Hmmm... where did you get those from?"

Her: "Topshop. Oh, I know! I'm going to take you shopping!" (At which point I start to panic).

"Now you've lost all this weight me and you will go to Cardiff and spend the day in Topshop. We'll get you some of that nice Kate Moss stuff, a little dress and a waistcoat with those big brass buttons on. And while we're at it we'll get you a fluorescent patterned top and some leggings. We can go round Bargoed looking like twins! Great, innit?"

I'm too much of a lady to respond to that, but it got me thinking about 'celebrity' clothes ranges, wondering if I'd be tempted to go to Evans to see what Fern Britton, or maybe Dawn French, would do with chiffon or stretch cotton.

Back to reality and imagining that Moss was one of my clothes idols (with a bit of back-combing and longer dresses I might consider it), I have to admit that I'm not a dedicated follower of fashion.

I'm – don't hate me for sounding poncy – too French for that.

Because the French buy what suits; they don't buy

what's 'in'.

Anyway, isn't it a little anachronistic to ask a model, with no technical design training, to make a range of clothes for the 'normal' woman?

Call me old-fashioned when it comes to fashion, but I thought a model's job was to make bad clothes look good.

For my money, buying into statement clothes or trends isn't a virtuous binge.

Frankly, I'd rather go it alone (but you don't really get 'unique' on sale in the places I shop, just more 'I'm dressing as a thin person but in a bigger size' tat, by and LARGE).

I just don't get why most people in this country have to have what's hot at the moment, which explains the abundance of Fame-like leggings, those flip-flopping shoes and low-slung trannie belts made out of old disc cutter blades.

So much nonsense surrounded the opening of the Kate Moss collection in Topshop, you'd have thought Glastonbury had come early or the Queen was in town.

With just a few hours to go until the range was launched at a special preview in London, people were starting to queue up outside, with every 150 given a different-coloured wrist-band.

Once the doors opened, only 150 people were allowed in at a time, with the numbers controlled by said bands.

They also received goodie bags with refreshments and booklets with a list of dos and don'ts once inside the store.

The latter included 'no more than five items per customer', and 'no items in multiple sizes' in an attempt to dissuade people from selling their goods on eBay; no more than 20 minutes' shopping time; 'no camera equipment in-store' and 'don't attempt to grapple, beg or bribe – you know you'll be embarrassed tomorrow'.

I, for one, won't be queuing up when Kate's clothes come to Wales today.

No, I'm waiting to be asked to design my own line for Evans called Reality (Big Bloody) Bites.

Can't see that making the headlines though, can you? I'd give out cakes instead of wristbands, so that everyone could be divided up by the colour of their favourite fondant fancies, and suggest smock tops worn over trousers.

Unlike Kate's, the hems wouldn't be so high that the world, to quote Patsy from Absolutely Fabulous, becomes your gynaecologist.

I'm not interested in buying something that makes Kate Moss look like, well, Kate Moss.

I'd camp out all night, though, for something that made me feel that I have it going on again.

But I've not yet heard of anyone getting Delusion in a size 24.

Life is tough enough without having someone kick you from the inside

Rita Rudner

SPOTTED: VICTORIA CAROLINE BECKHAM at La Noisette in Sloane Street, SW1, feasting – ha! – on a green salad without olive oil, steamed red mullet, steamed veg and a fruit plate.

And you wonder how she stays a zero hero, eh?

Caught: Hannah Marie Jones in the passage of her terraced house secretly stuffing a ham sandwich while waiting for her eggs (four) to boil to make a salad, a packet of salt'n'vinegar crisps, two yoghurts, a banana, a punnet of strawberries, three oranges and a bag of black grapes.

I knew something was up when fruit came into the equation.

I thought, you see, I was pregnant.

It didn't take a lot to convince me, if you count the fruit craving shocker and a period that was an hour or something late.

So forgive me for thinking I was with child because I suddenly fancied fruit and not coal-topped ice-cream, gherkin sarnies or mayo on toast.

But it wasn't to be.

Significant (thin) Other, the know-it-all star-gazer of my life, said I was run down (I was) and that my body was having a vitamin C 'craving', whatever the hell that is.

"What, like I normally crave a cheese, ham and

mushroom pizza from Jeff's Pizza Pan in Ebbw Vale when I'm on a diet you mean?" came my confused reply, not quite getting the I MUST HAVE FRUIT NOW thing.

"Yeah, just like that," he told me, slowly. "People can crave fruit too, you know."

At that I laughed in his beautiful face – granted, while picking pips out of my teeth – because I was sure I was about to start choosing baby clothes in my head.

It didn't take me long to start imagining names you could safely shout at when buying your Tampax at Tesco – "Oi, Truly Scrumptious Beaufort Belle, come back 'ere now!" doesn't really cut it if you want to go unnoticed in a crisis – and revelling in the idea that for nine months I could eat for two.

Or 222 in my case (I was always shit at counting, my excuse for failing at keeping tabs on calories too).

I wasn't even worried about getting back in shape after the birth.

After all, round's a shape, right?

Size, don't you know, has superseded sex as the subject that we love to talk about.

So, by my unreasonable reasoning, I could opt out of the cool craze if I found myself in maternity gear, lulled into a false sense of security by the thought of elastic on EVERYTHING.

Happy in the haze of a potential eater's paradise, with the promise of a rosy-cheeked Mini-Me popping out of me instead of confusion, I started to do a bit of research on the web, trying to find out where I could get kitted out.

I also wanted to see if any other biggies had written stuff about being pregnant and large.

I was curious about this because, in my phantom pregnant life, I was really scared of going to the doctor.

That's because I've always been made to feel that ANYTHING that's wrong with me is the result of being overweight.

In-growing toenail? *"Have you thought about going on a diet?"*

Throat infection? *"Here you are, have some nice leaflets on diets which could help you."*

Contraception? *"You don't need it if you're fat, surely. There's nothing safer than blubber, girl!"*

Cold sores? *"There's tablets you can take to help you lose weight. Want to go on them AGAIN?"*

Bad knee? *"There's lots of pressure on your joints, obviously. Frankly love, I wouldn't want to be your cartilage if you know what I mean."*

Simultaneous sneeze-n-wee problems? *"I could prescribe a commode for you so you can sit on it while you're watching an episode of The Vicar of Dibley."*

Irregular and heavy periods? *"It's obvious why that's going on. You're FAT FAT FAT!"*

And, surprise surprise, I stumbled on a report which said that fat pregnant women are a burden on the NHS.

A study found that obese pregnant women need more one-to-one care, which can have an impact on waiting times for other patients.

Bigger women are also more likely to need extra scans and tests, have more caesarean deliveries, need more specialist equipment and have less choice when it comes to giving birth than other girls.

They suffer higher rates of infection, can need extra support with breastfeeding, and there are added risks for the baby. Or so they say.

The pros complain that the trolleys aren't big enough for them, longer needles are needed for spinal anaesthesia and nurses take extra time to prepare additional equipment to hold fat back during Caesarean sections.

Nice, eh?

Doctors can't even let you glow for a moment without highlighting the fact that your impending expansion on your expanse pisses everyone off.

So not only are we excluded from the mainstream shops, we're also made to feel like second-class citizens at the doctor's.

But big girls are natural rebels. The cool pregnant big girl doesn't give a damn, though.

She's all about living in the moment, celebrating her bumps and folds.

She's a happy-eyed Mother Earth type, a beautiful little sauce-pot who will accentuate the positives about being big and bountifully pregnant.

Thinnies, look on and weep. You may have more choice when it comes to maternity clothes, but at least we're assured of one thing – and that's knowing that you never, *ever,* see an ugly fat baby. Well, do you?

Maybe that's because its mother ate enough cake to keep it happy way before this big bad world decided to make her feel guilty about having it near her mouth in the first place.

> # If you get melted chocolate all over your hands, you're eating it too slowly
>
> **Anonymous**

I'D BEEN CONTEMPLATING MY dieting future with a packet of Deep Ridge (max flavour you understand) crisps.

Paprika ones, just so you can get the full picture.

I'd spent my entire lunch hour thinking about my body while nibbling on an egg mayonnaise sandwich.

Sorry, let me rephrase that – it wasn't a lunch hour per se. It was 9.30. in the morning (supper at that time would be just plain wrong. But I have dabbled on the dark side). I washed my musings down with a semi-skimmed latte to go (small), and tin of pineapple chunks (my one nod to the 5-a-day demands).

I think there were about three boiled eggs in there too, and a pinch of anxiety, although I can't be certain of anything right now. I'm in a daze, see. And not one caused by a sugar rush.

For a few weeks, I've been in early-morning, mid-afternoon and late-night quandaries about being categorically useless.

I was convinced at the end of my mental digestions that if someone cut me in half – if they found a chain saw big enough that is – they'd see the words 'can't stick to anything' running through me.

I hadn't, you see, been going to diet class. Then it got worse. A story I had to, ahem, research for the Magazine I edit saw me being sent 10 giant cakes, made to make sure you could really taste the difference.

Their tempting and sudden presence in my life ensured my position in that mental state of dieters everywhere, called a downer.

I already wasn't watching my calories, didn't care what I felt like and generally just couldn't be arsed with the general show of denying myself a slice (well, 50 at least if nobody had been watching) of the taste-to-die-for good life.

So they came in. And I ate. I also shared. I didn't think twice as everyone else was digging in. So I had some more.

I did a bit of exercise in the night to make up for over-indulging, then had another bite of something to congratulate myself, pretending I was conducting some quality 'research' in the name of product testing (I don't think I was supposed to swallow though).

You know the drill.

Then just as I was regaining interest in myself, reminding my inner demons that just a few weeks ago I had been a sliver off a two-stone loss, some Ignorant Bugger brought me down even further.

The truncated version is that I said something funny, someone else thought to come back with a witty retort (don't try this at home, I'm razor-tongued, me), then IB, trying to be a smart-arse goes, "I wouldn't say that to her (i.e. me) as I'm scared of her. She's much too big to argue with. Watch it or she'll crush you with more than her tongue!"

Hmmm. Do you think he meant I am an intellectual giant? Tall? Important in the office hierarchy?

Fat injected chance.

I don't know what it is about me that makes people think that they can say ANYTHING to me and I'll just shrug it off.

Perhaps I come across as someone who doesn't have any hang-ups, who isn't bothered about how I look or how I'm perceived; a walking, talking, bundle of steel who is immune to jibes, however innocently intentioned.

Get this everyone: I'M NOT A FAT JOAN RIVERS.

So I did what any good crashing dieter does, I had cake. Then more cake. Then cake on top of the cake. And topped it off not with cherries (I don't understand why anyone ruins a good treat with fruit – what the hell is pineapple on a pizza about?) but more cake.

And do you know the worst thing of all? I've never been big – oi, no sniggering from the cheap seats – on cake.

Corned beef rolls are more my nose bag, but needs must, you know?

Anyway, the good news is that I returned to Fat Club last Monday and I think/hope/pray I'm back on track.

As long as I don't have to do a story on homemade quiche, I think next week's going to be OK.

> **I don't have a problem with my body. I don't diet, and I'm not hiding anything. I'm not going to be the subject of a movie of the week 10 years from now**
>
> **Lara Flynn Boyle**

"BLOODY HELL, SHE'S A porker, isn't she," Steve said. Steve, still with a fake tan only going up one arm (the cheap shop had run out so he couldn't do the other one), used the same description to talk about two girls this week.

The first time he used it, he was describing Wangers, the Welsh contestant on Big Brother.

Pal Tanners went on to say that new girl Wangers, a fellow advocate of gravy browning your skin, was "even bigger than you" meaning Me, if you're following my drift, a backhanded compliment if ever I heard one.

And then it became complicated.

I'm plus-sized, she's just plus-breasted. There is a difference.

I tried explaining this concept to Tan Hands in simple terms, but nothing would assuage him.

I like Laura aka Wangers; I like the fact she loves drinking squash, hates fags and describes herself as "happy, happy, happy".

It makes her quirky, honest and great entertainment.

It now also makes her, because her oven mitts are more than average, open to being labelled as a buxom, big-boned, bountiful fat bird.

Let me repeat again – SHE'S NOT FAT SHE'S JUST

274

RICH IN THRUP'NY BITS.

They make her look top heavy, yes; but this doesn't mean she's shopping in Elvi for her leggings and pink belts.

A bit of back combing, looser clothes and an up-top minimiser, and the evidence would out.

Trust me, I'm a journalist.

It makes me sad, though, that people around the country will invariably refer to her as "that fat Welsh one with the huge tits" when discussing the crazy clubhouse that is Big Brother.

Already I'm hearing rumours that our girl is the favourite to win, her unpretentiousness, cheery manner and earthiness already proving popular.

But then web sites started popping up musing on her ability to stay sane in the madhouse.

And why? Because insensitive webheads are taking bets on if she'll have a nervous breakdown because – get this – she's the least pretty and one of the 'fattest' in there.

Nice, eh? Do they think that someone that happy, that content, that nice gives a shit about not feeling up to par with some of the other vacuous fashion victims she's sharing that place with?

I bet she's doesn't give a Wangers.

Then came the second "Bloody hell, she's a porker, isn't she" musings from Brown Boy I'd Better Not Go In The Rain.

This time he was referring to a copy of the NME I was reading, the one where 'fat' singing pin-up Beth Ditto was pictured naked.

She looked, well, fat. But she's got more balls than me.

Beth, though, doesn't care about taking her clothes

off, or wearing stuff more suitable for a size 8.

I don't quite get that, don't understand why such a big girl feels the needs to parade around in tight clothes even a stick insect wouldn't be caught in.

But you've got to give her credit for exposing a body that the world, certainly the fashion industry and glossy magazines, thinks should be kept hidden.

It makes me want to stick out my not inconsiderable chest, tousle up my hair, paint my lips blood-red and let someone take a picture of me eating a juicy red apple, like some Wicked Witch of the Fridge.

Then I'd suggest a group shot with Wangers, Beth, Fern, Dawn, Jo, Roseanne and me.

We'd call it The Naked Truth: Big Girls Let It All Hang Out.

And I'd defy anybody to call this little lot porkers.

Because the fall out (ahem) would be worth its considerable weight in BOLD.

> **I have gained and lost the same ten pounds so many times over and over again my cellulite must have déjà vu**
>
> **Jane Wagner**

I RECEIVED THIS LETTER the other day.

Dear Hannah,
I just wanted to drop you a line to say how much I am enjoying your 'Diary of a Diet' column.

I have been reading it every week, but this week's one was really fantastic.

I am going to a diet class at the moment after the nurse at my doctor's surgery told me I was fat. Your column really captures the atmosphere (and frustration) of slimming classes.

I have had an extra 'naughty' weekend (I'm talking Domino's pizza, fish and chips and bacon, not salad) and know I have to face the scales on Thursday feeling the same way you did.

So thank you for making me smile and not feel quite so guilty about my sure-to-be-terrible weigh-in.

It really is a great read.

I know who sent me this and I don't think she's over a size 14. She's also nice and tall, so I guess her BMI, that crazy chart which tells the pros if we're fine, or fat, or flipping-hell-you-need-to-sew-up-your-gob enormous, wouldn't be in the danger zone.

Aside from the fact that I sighed at this lovely young thing being told she was a slab of meat by some know-all holding a blood pressure machine, it was good to read that my 24-sized struggles are similar to those who I would consider normal.

Then I got this one.

Dear Inflated Plastic Valleys Girl Editor,

I don't know who you think you are, but I, for one, think you're self-indulgent, crass, ignorant and, face facts love, you're also FAT!

You think you're talking for every woman out there who can't lose weight? You're not.

Let me tell you something for nothing, you don't speak for me.

You, like every other woman on a diet out there, are useless at it but you still keep on doing it. You don't succeed, yet you still make a living out of moaning about it.

Know what you want? You want to eat less and run more!

Simple as. So I suggest you get up off your fat arse and spend the time you would normally spend writing this crap jogging around the park.

Oh, do you think I hit a nerve?

Anyway, I laughed out loud at the Inflated Plastic Valleys Girl tag.

I had visions of myself in the Chinese, my new pair of fake breasts stuffed into a red swimming costume, blonde hair topped off with a nice Dai Cap.

Then the image of Dawn French running in that French and Saunders Baywatch skit entered my head and my bubble was well and truly burst.

I find it amazing that:

a. I can wind people up like this;

b. Slim girls crash diet;

c. I cause such diverse and discordant reactions.

The other day I went shopping with someone in their 50s who has been on a diet for 49 years.

She's always on one eating plan or another, always struggling to be smaller than she is, but bigger in every other way, like dropping a few dress sizes will somehow increase her personal power.

So I said to her, why not stop? Why not think that now, aged 50-odd, it was time to accept herself for who and what she is.

She looked at me like I had two heads on my Inflated Plastic Valleys Girl shoulders and said, "Because it's not what I do. I diet. I moan about it. I lose weight. I don't. I get depressed. I think bugger it. I start all over again. Have you tried the pineapple and ham fat plan, Han? I might give that a go to see if it does it for me this time."

My friend doesn't read this column so she isn't inspired by it; by that reasoning, she also can't hate it.

She doesn't have an opinion about it because she's too busy having negative ones about herself.

And when she loses some weight, they magically blossom into glorious positive ones.

So to all you dieters out there, I've one piece of advice to you: Ignore your detractors and just get on with doing your own thing – even if you'll never be a Baywatch babe, you can still look good ordering dim sum to go.

I AM, DON'T YOU know it, an inspiration. Hi, Han fans!

On the train into work the other day I was spotted by someone who recognised me, not from my work as an extra on the Thriller video (I wasn't having a very good hair/belly day), but from my by-line picture at the top of the page where my column sits.

Anyway, this beautiful stranger said she'd gone back to Fat Club because she was inspired by me to take the plunge against the bulge once again.

Honest to God, that's what she said.

Through reading this column she felt spurred on and invigorated because I'd made the American in her mind come out of hibernation, high-fiving itself and shouting "You can do it girl! You have it going ON!" for the first time in, oh, what was it now? That's right, yep, a month.

She hadn't been 'off it' for long, just enough time to feel like shit and put some weight back on.

But not any more. No, apparently the story of Jesus Jones, the one who kept the five loaves for herself, had made her feel that this time she was going to win the dieting fight and get down to a 'reasonable' size 14.

Luckily, she could do enough talking for the both of us because at that point I was just sitting there with my mouth open.

And no, I wasn't just stretching the muscles so that my face wouldn't go into involuntary spasm with the heavenly shock of eating two cheese topped rolls after

280

weeks of calorie counting and dairy dodging.

"Me? I've spurred you on to go back on your diet? I'm bloody useless!" was my honest response.

"No, you're doing really, really, really well and I think you inspire loads of women out there," said my new best friend, who was being sainted for Services to Those With Special Bread Needs in the Community that afternoon, I think.

Ah, the big are sometimes so dumb. We'll reach out for anything in our hour of need (usually crisps or a sorry tale from a fellow blob-battler whose sob story – and thighs, as they'll always look out for this one – are bigger than their own).

I didn't tell her, but I frankly find the idea of sailing home from Turkey on a pedalo easier to believe than that I'm a model of good behaviour.

This is because the last two weeks have been dreadful, dietary-wise.

It all started to go horribly wrong when, at lunchtime, I waved off the thinnies from the office as they headed in the direction of Dorothy Perkins for a 20% off shopping spree.

They went off en masse while I stayed manning the phones, nibbling on resentment for my lunch and stewing in my own jealousy juices for afters (I think the old-fashioned methods of losing weight are sometimes the most effective, don't you?).

I managed to fit in a lot of angst while they fitted themselves out in new summer clothes.

Honestly, I must have looked pitiful waving them off on their voyage into High Street bargain land.

It's a mystical place which I've never seen, as no biggie can find it, even with the use of a personal shopper, as we're all denied entry by virtue of the fact that we can hide a child under our bellies and do star jumps without it moving an inch.

That was 14 days ago and since then I've forgotten to remember to be good. My uncanny ability to find an M&S food hall anywhere in the country, while blindfolded, hasn't deserted me, however.

I've had what I'd call a nutritional melt-down and lost interest in watching what I nibbled.

After all, a DP's discount day felt like a hell of a lot of missed lunches away.

So why miss them, right?

The only good behaviour I've been involved in lately was washing the butter knife before I put it in garlic mayonnaise while making chicken and sweetcorn rolls (two, crusty, just to ensure my rightful place in culinary hell).

Svelte Stranger, bless her heart, said that the reason she'd stopped going to get weighed THE MOST RECENT TIME (she's been on a diet for 27 years, apparently), was that she was fed up waking up and thinking about food every second of the day – what she could eat, what she couldn't put in her mouth, what not to mix together in case she blew up, or at least blow off in public.

But for some reason, my story had spurred her into action once again, and she was now ready to go back to being obsessed by food. And all because of me.

"Why do it again if it made you so unhappy the last time?" I asked her. "You're telling me that you're going to go back to thinking about food all the time."

"Yeah," she said. "You do it and you've lost two stone. You're an (there's that word again) inspiration (bollocks!) to us all."

At times like these, days where any unguarded

emotion leaves me wanting to do that dreaded inedible dieting faux pas – go late night food shopping when I'm hungry – hairline cracks start to appear in my resolve.

I become unresponsive to common sense, feeling a pound of fat away from being cited by the BMI Police as uncommunicative and weak around fridges.

That's inspirational? Is it hell.

The trouble with professional dieters like me and the lovely train traveller, those who yo-yo like billy-oh, is twofold, as I see it – we've failed because of our inability to stay motivated and stay interested in the notion of our better selves.

We lose weight for a bit and by doing so we think – delusionally – we're starting to get some clarity.

And what happens then, when we sniff out a bit of personal success?

Colours become brighter, our sense of smell intensifies, we start to think we can walk on heels let alone water.

And – here's the absolute clincher – food starts to taste better than ever before.

Isn't it ironic? Like your numbers coming up on the lottery and the promoter going bust the next morning. Or a no-smoking sign on your cigarette break. Thanks Alanis.

When it happens, after a sufficient period of time, we get fatter than we were in the first place and the cycle starts again.

Notice I didn't say 'cycling' there.

Now that really would be something poignant.

> **I told my doctor I get very tired when I go on a diet, so he gave me pep pills. Know what happened? I ate faster**
>
> Joe E. Lewis

I PUT ON THREE and a half pounds last week. Did you catch that?

It took all my inner might and gentle cajoling from those with my best interests at heart to go back to Fat Club after a three-week hiatus.

I knew what was coming, right?

I knew that I'd go in, have to line-up with the majority of thin fat-loathers who scream out at their half-pound loss – "I can't believe it! And I've been really, really bad at the weekend – nibbling on two nuts, sucking an olive and having three chips on my dinner of air" – then have to smile at their joyousness.

It's what you do, another unwritten rule of attendance that's up there with Thou Shall Not Mix Carbs And Proteins Together and Look In The Mirror Twice A Day To Remind Yourself Why You're Here You Fat Cow.

You share dessert. Oops, butter fingers, I mean delight (but not of the Angel variety, sadly).

If you think you've seen ecstasy on someone's face before, think again.

Take my word for it, if you want to see real euphoria in action, find a slimming class and prepare to watch grown women scream like kids on Christmas day when they've lost a little weight.

They can't contain their excitement as the jeans which

contain their bellies miraculously get that little bit looser as they step off the scales.

Where I'm from, it always happens between 6.30p.m. and 8p.m. on a Monday.

I've seen tears of joy at a one pound loss, whoops for two pounds, high-pitched screams only a dog could hear at three pounds, the can-can round the room with the mention of five pounds gone, and sheer euphoria if more than that has disappeared into the twilight zone.

But as they all – bar none – were congratulating themselves for not eating much for seven days on the trot, yours truly was secretly being demoted from Slimmer of the Week (four times) to Full-Fat Prat.

You know that thing people do when they describe a big person? They shrug their shoulders and puff out their arms, extend the old elbows, form fists and clench. Know the one?

Well I had that when I went back to class.

There I was, last but one in line to receive the digitally-enhanced bad news of my dieting reality.

I was talking to a size 12 who'd lost the not-so-grand total of three pounds in five weeks in her bid to wear a size 8, telling her not to give up hope as I'd lost two stone so far.

And if I can do it, anyone can blah, blah, ugh and ah.

She'd sounded deflated, see. And I, trying not to shout in her face "You stupid bitch, how small do you want to be?!", tried to play the encouragement card in the (scrawny, cheekbone-hugging) face of her despondency.

So I told her I was bound to put on weight as I hadn't been for three weeks, but that I hadn't given up hope.

I'd just put it on the back-burner for a little while, that's all.

Our conflab started out nicely enough.

"I'm going out for a meal later and I've been saving up all my calories for five garlic mushrooms and one half of a crusty roll," she confided.

"God, I hope I've lost as I'll have to limit myself to four if I haven't."

Then she turned into Thinzilla.

"How much did you say you'd lost?"

(It was two stone before I'd gone off the boil and back to egg-fried rice.)

"Don't suppose anyone's noticed, have they? It must be hard being such a big (shrug, puff, extend, fist and clench: copyright Jones) girl like you," she threw at me.

"Because I'm small, anything I lose is bound to show up really quickly. People will notice.

"Whereas you, because you're so big (and repeat the move as necessary) will have to lose stones upon stones before anyone will notice the difference.

"But at least you're on the right track. Loads to go though!

"It must be very frustrating for you."

It is; and no, I didn't tell her it was.

Anyway, I didn't have a chance. As I was preparing my speech, my "You may be thin but you're also ugly which makes me wonder if people go dressed up as you at Halloween" jibe, she was called up to weigh in.

What followed could only be described as orgasmic, her "Yes! Yes! Yes!" belted out in ecstatic abandon.

Because she'd lost seven pounds, that slimming holy grail which says you're on the right track.

The Queen of the Slimmers, the Fat Club VIP, received a rapturous round of applause from every hopeful dieter in the class, those who'd broken the pound barrier and others who live perpetually in the land of hope.

My reversal of fortune, my tumble from grace, my inability not to fall into the descriptive shoulder-shrugging range is totally my own fault.

I'd wanted an extra piece of fresh cream sponge AND a third crusty ham roll AND another ice cream AND a second pizza slice AND Sunday sinner (sic) on a Monday.

And I'd put on three and a half pounds.

It really is as shoulder-shruggingly, fist-clenchingly, heart-breakingly simple as that.

> **I've been on a constant diet for the last two decades. I've lost a total of 789 pounds. By all accounts, I should be hanging from a charm bracelet**
>
> **Erma Bombeck**

20ST 2LB.THAT'S WHAT it says on the first page of my Fat Club book.

18st 1lb. That's what the latest entry has me at.

Actually it only says that on the scales in Boots where I'm always four pounds lighter, so I'm often popping in there to play fantasy weights.

Nobody believes I weigh that much, as heavy as a rugby player with a better choice in shoes (then again…).

But that's what it says, straight up, no messing around, no exaggeration, no squinting through one eye or breathing in when I step on the scales.

At the start of this book, I made a point of not telling you what I weighed, primarily because I didn't want to do to the thinnies what the fashion world, short-sighted fellas and society have been doing to us buxom babes for years – alienate them.

Five months on from that first Fat Club weigh-in, but an age since I first started the 'Diary of a Diet' column in the I – to say nothing of the 30-year anniversary of first hearing the words, "Don't worry, you'll lose your puppy fat when you're 16… Now please, *PLEASE* step away from that beef and onion roll!" – and I'm still cheating, still not attending class on a regular basis (I lasted three months before I got fed up of weighing out cheese), still binging, still struggling, still feeling amazed at the times when I'm not.

I'm wondering if my love of basic foods and dissatisfaction with the way I am (read: look) isn't really a sign that there's something much bigger that is eating at me (sadly it's not a tape worm chomping on my wobbly bits).

I'm here, trying to coax my bad habits out of me one cheesecake refusal at a time.

I am not a dieting success story, despite losing two stone. If I was focused, committed, stronger than I am, I could be well on the way to a five-stone loss. You know it, and I know it too.

But I'm trying to be as good as I can so that, on the more frequent occasions that I'm Bad Hannah, I can pick myself up a little bit quicker.

It works – occasionally. The trick, for me, is coming to terms with the awful realisation that it doesn't work as often as I'd like it to and that I'm not as good as I dream I could be.

It's shit I know – but not as shit as Pizza Hut not having drive-thrus in the UK when you haven't done your hair and you can't be arsed to wait.

Some things you've just got to learn to live with.

To change the way I live my life would be to alter the basic essence of me.

I am, and have always been, someone who defines themselves by how they deal with their 'issues'; someone who rallies against being seen as pale and inward-looking.

Maybe this kind of thinking is crap and pathetic, but it's the only reasoning I know.

When I set about compiling all my columns together for this *Little Book of Big*, as well as tap out some more slim musings on my bloody big life, I really wanted this to be a story with which most women could relate to.

Fat or thin, deluded or not.

Whether I have succeeded, of course, is your call.

I've also realised that if I pick up that extra large pizza for one after a week of salads, and then drive ten miles so nobody who has my best interests at heart can see me dispose of the box, it's mine.

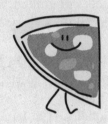

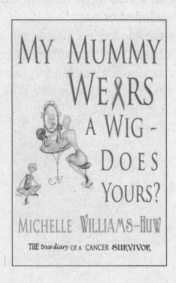

A true and heart-warming account of a journey through breast cancer.

A diagnosis of breast cancer made Michelle Williams-Huw, mother of two small boys, re-evaluate her life as she battled her demons to come to terms with the illness. *My Mummy Wears A Wig* is poignant, sad, revelatory and deliciously funny. Readers will be riveted by her honesty and enchanted as, having hit bottom, she falls in love with life (and her husband) all over again.

ISBN 9781906125110   price £7.99

Laughing All Over The World

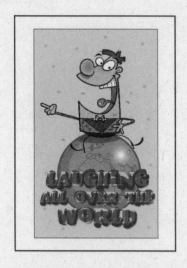

FOREWORD by PENELOPE KEITH

With contributions from: Stephen Fry,
Tom Stoppard, Richard Briers, Tim Brooke-Taylor,
Dom Wood, Arthur Smith, Sara Cox, Niamh
Cusack and Jim Sweeney.

A unique full-colour cartoon and joke book for all the family.

Children, celebrities, comedians and cartoonists from the UK and overseas have contributed rib-ticklers, one-liners, anecdotes and cartoons to this incredible compendium of fun. Ideal for all the family, this book is destined to fill a multitude of stockings this year.

ISBN – 9781906125059 price £5.99